Once you enter, you will not emerge the
same . . .

IN THE DEEP WOODS

NICHOLAS CONDÉ is the author of *The Religion*
(the basis for the film *The Believers*) and *The Leg-
end*. He lives in New York City.

IN THE DEEP WOODS

NICHOLAS CONDÉ

ST. MARTIN'S PRESS / NEW YORK

Grateful acknowledgement is made to the following for permission to reprint from previously published material:

Williamson Music Co. for lyrics from "It Might as Well Be Spring" by Richard Rodgers and Oscar Hammerstein II. Copyright © 1945 by Williamson Music Co. Used by permission. All rights reserved.

Robbins Music Corporation for lyrics from "I'm in the Mood for Love" by Dorothy Fields and Jimmy McHugh. Copyright © 1935 (Renewed 1963) Robbins Music Corporation. All rights of Robbins Music Corporation assigned to SBK Catalogue Partnership. All rights controlled and administered by SBK Robbins Catalog Inc. International Copyright secured. All rights reserved.

Revelation Music Publishing Corp. & Rilting Music, Inc. for: Lyrical excerpts from "Ballad of Sweeney Todd." Music and lyrics by Stephen Sondheim. Copyright © 1979 Revelation Music Publishing Corp. & Rilting Music, Inc. A Tommy Valando Publication.

IN THE DEEP WOODS

Copyright © 1989 by Nicholas Condé.

Library of Congress Catalog Card Number: 88-30539

ISBN 0-312-92094-6   Can. ISBN: 0-312-92095-4

Printed in the United States of America

St. Martin's Press hardcover edition published 1989
First St. Martin's Press mass market edition / March 1990

10 9 8 7 6 5 4 3 2 1

For all the crew aboard *Breakaway*

Little children do not like it when there is talk of the inborn human inclination to "badness," and to aggressiveness and destructiveness and cruelty as well. For God has made children in the image of His own perfection, and no one wants to be reminded how hard it is to reconcile His all-powerfulness and His all-goodness with the undeniable existence of evil.

—Sigmund Freud
Civilization and Its Discontents

IN THE
DEEP
WOODS

Maybe it had something to do with phases of the moon.

No, he thought, and laughed quietly to himself, he wasn't a werewolf. No fangs surging from between his lips, no claws suddenly sprouting from his hands. Just the urge, arriving in his mind with no warning, no more fanfare than a letter being dropped through a mail slot.

As always, during the moments when he had to wait quietly, he couldn't help wondering about it—the trigger. What was it? In all the years he'd lived with these eruptions of need, he had never been able to pin down any specific catalyst. They had come upon him in so many different circumstances. After a good meal at a roadside diner, or on a sunny weekend afternoon when he finished fixing a leaky kitchen faucet, and once, he remembered, after waking at two in the morning to chase a sparrow that had flown in through the hall window. Always the same, he thought. One moment he would be concerned only with the banal business of a normal day, and then he would find himself launched again on one of these . . . these quests.

Warding off the chill of the October night, he flipped up the collar of his sport jacket, then glanced at his watch. This was the part he always liked, even relished—the waiting, the building of anticipation for the challenge to come . . . yet he was uncomfortable in the cold. He should have taken a scarf, he scolded himself mildly, or a sweater. He always tried to cling too long to the conveniences of warmer weather. Wearing less meant less to lose. A scarf would be just one more thing to keep track of, one more potential problem.

He whistled a bar of a song and tried for a second to remember the title, then a snatch of the lyric came to his lips. "I'm as jumpy as a puppet on a string . . . ," and he finished the line quietly in his mind: *"I'd say that I had spring fever, but I know it isn't spring."* He smiled at the irony; the urge was strong, but he never felt particularly feverish, and certainly not jumpy. The feeling was more of being caught up by . . . by what? A mission, he thought, even a duty.

The smile vanished abruptly from his lips and his mind stopped its ramblings as the shadowy figure of a lone young woman emerged from a doorway of the building on the other side of the parking lot. She began to walk across the broad asphalt field, past the few remaining cars toward another cluster of buildings.

As he prepared to step from his shadowy waiting place, he felt a rush of fresh energy. He took a deep breath, filling his lungs the way a champion swimmer did when poised at the edge of the water in the last moment before diving into the race.

It was more difficult to walk than he had anticipated, and he had to hurry the last ten yards. The extra effort made him breathe a little faster, and he knew that wasn't good. He had to seem casual, relaxed. That was the key.

And when the crucial moment arrived, he did it beautifully, every move performed exactly as planned.

The pretty young woman turned, aware of him for the first time, and peered through the narrow span of darkness that separated them.

That pause for a sensible assessment . . . it was almost always the same. Reassured, she took a step closer. He concentrated on gathering up the things he had dropped, pretending not to notice.

At last, all doubt dispelled, she spoke the necessary, perfect question.

"Would you like some help?"

Only then did he look up and give her a smile so nice that, even veiled by the chill dark, it struck the girl as dazzling. . . .

1 "RANDY," THE LITTLE GIRL SAID. She moved up to the head of the line and handed over the book. "It's for me, so you can write it. 'To Randy.' "

Carol Warren no sooner poised her pen to write an inscription than the stocky, severe woman beside the little girl leaned over and amended the instructions. "Her name's Miranda. Write it 'To Miranda,' I'd prefer that."

Carol hesitated. Why shouldn't the name be written exactly as the child had asked? The book was going to belong to her, wasn't it?

But the moment seemed wrong for giving parental advice. In front of the oversize rocking chair where authors sat while signing books at The Friendly Giant bookstore, five other children-with-mothers were already waiting to get *In the Dragon's Cave* autographed by its author-illustrator.

"To Miranda," Carol duly wrote in the flowery script she used on these occasions, "love 'n' lollipops, Carol Warren."

The little girl accepted the book with a grateful smile.

"Why do you want to be called Randy?" the mother could be heard carping as they moved off. "That's a boy's name. . . ."

After the next five children came a break in the stream of buyers. The frail, balding young man who owned The Friendly Giant had been standing near Carol at the side of the rear alcove called The Author's

Corner. "This is a wonderful turnout," he said, leaning toward her. "We haven't done this well since Sendak was here."

"I'm glad you're pleased," Carol said.

"More than pleased. If it keeps up this way, we'll sell a hundred copies." He glanced at his watch. "While there's a lull I'd be happy to buy you lunch. You've been at it two hours."

Carol had already sensed his interest in her and suspected that the invitation to lunch meant something more. She felt a twinge of guilt in discouraging him. "Thanks, but I'd better stay here," she said with her warmest smile. "If anyone else shows up, I wouldn't want to keep them waiting."

Which was the truth. Carol was sincerely grateful to the children who showed enthusiasm for her work. It wasn't so long ago that a bookstore would announce her appearance to sign books and no one would show up. But then came Christmas four years ago—and publication of *Dana's Dark Ocean,* Carol's fantasy about a sea monster who befriends a fisherman's daughter. The book had been a surprise best-seller, and since then all of Carol's books had sold in steadily increasing numbers.

The line for autographs began to form again. Brief as the respite had been, it had broken the rhythm of automatic signing, and Carol again took time to chat a little with each child as she had earlier in the morning. With her fine features and fair complexion, slim build, and long pale blond hair swept back on either side with matching combs, Carol had a head start in friendship with any book-loving child—since she conformed to their notion of how the delicate yet spunky heroine of *Alice in Wonderland* must have looked. Not unaware of this quality, Carol sometimes played it up—especially at book signings—by wearing high-necked blouses rather than sophisticated dresses. She had, in fact, an air of unspoiled innocence that no

doubt explained why children not only appreciated
her work, but once they had met her in person were
quickly smitten. It accounted, too, for the fact that she
was extremely attractive to men, but at the same time
daunting. She gave the impression of holding her pas-
sions closely in check, of believing in one of the principal fantasies nurtured by her own profession—that the
Sleeping Beauty might only be awakened someday by
a special Prince Charming.

Carol had signed a dozen more books when she
looked up and saw not a child but a tall, stern-faced
man, eyeing her intensely.

There was something instantly unsettling about
him. Although adults often brought books to be autographed for children and grandchildren, the peculiar
way this man so firmly planted himself in front of
Carol gave her the feeling that his business wasn't so
simple or benign. He wore a dark serge overcoat that
looked too heavy for the early-autumn weather, and
a pearl-grey homburg tilted slightly forward so that his
eyes were partly in shadow. He didn't immediately
hold the book out, but kept it pressed flat against his
body, all but hidden in the grip of his large hands,
while he continued staring at her. It was almost as
though he were trying to make an identification, Carol
thought, matching her face to features he'd seen in a
written description.

Did he know her? She had a vague sense of recognition herself, as if she might recently have glimpsed
him somewhere—in a busy restaurant, or through a
gap on a crowded bus.

For a second or two she met the challenge of his
eyes with her own direct gaze. No, she didn't know
him, she was sure. But as her eyes lingered, she imagined how she might draw the face beneath the curled
brim of the homburg. His features were subtly shaped,
with high cheekbones creating an almost ascetic cast—
though if not carefully sketched, the large nose, broad

mouth, and deeply cleft chin might give a surly, un-sympathetic appearance. As imposing as he was, the overall effect was softened by his warm hazel eyes, marked at the corners with deep crinkles that suggested many days of squinting at the sun. His age was hard to judge—a few years either side of fifty, she thought. The hat and coat seemed the choice of an older man, but his erect stance and the fit of his clothes indicated strength and vigor. It was as if a grizzled ranch hand or logger had put on the costume of the city.

At last, unwilling to continue the duel of gazes, Carol put out her hand for the book. "Can I sign that for you . . . ?"

He passed it to her. "Thank you, Miss Warren, if you would."

She took note of his choice of words: genteel. And the voice: firm and resonant, but well-modulated—the voice of a man who had his strength under control. "And how would you like it inscribed?" she asked, opening the book.

He regarded her skeptically—as if he thought she should know what he wanted without asking.

Then he said, "Make it 'To Suzanne,' please—with a z."

At another time Carol might have asked if "Suzanne" was a grandchild or drawn out some fact to personalize the inscription. But a stricken look flaring in the man's eyes hinted at some deep emotion behind his request, and Carol was suddenly anxious for the encounter to end.

To Suzanne, she dashed off in her everyday handwriting, *Best wishes, Carol Warren.*

She thrust the book back at him and offered only a tight smile before pointedly turning to the little boy next in line and extending her hand. "Hello, what's your name?"

As she wrote a new inscription, Carol was aware of

the dark overcoat moving out of her field of vision, and she couldn't resist looking up to make sure he had left. In the aisles between her and the door the man was nowhere in sight.

For a while after he had left, Carol found her thoughts returning to him whenever the line of buyers tapered off. But as the afternoon went on, so many other faces came past her that even the most unusual was no longer isolated in her memory. The man in the homburg was merely someone who had decided to buy a book, a man odd enough to make a brief impression, but not someone she was ever likely to see again.

Carol arrived home at a little past six o'clock. Kicking off her shoes as she came in, she went to the kitchen, took an unfinished bottle of white wine from the refrigerator, and poured herself a glass. She carried it back to the living room, tuned the stereo to WQXR, and flopped onto the couch.

Pleased with the day's accomplishment—the final tally of books sold was 128—she felt like celebrating a little. For a second she wondered if she'd been too hasty in declining the bookstore owner's second invitation, to have supper with him. It might have made a nice end to the day, but as she stretched out on the couch Carol reconfirmed her decision. She had spent time enough with the sweet but reticent young man to know a date would have led nowhere. Another dead-end evening, pleasant but meaningless conversation, a groping attempt to make a deeper connection that would end with his asking for another date and her making excuses. God, how many times she'd been through it . . .

Sipping her wine, Carol reflected on the period after her breakup with Richard, when she had made a determined effort not to become a recluse, to date, to accept dinner invitations from friends even though she knew she'd be seated next to a "most eligible

bachelor" type. None of it had really worked out. Was
she too hard to please? No, after two and a half years
of living with Richard Caldwell, it was inevitable that
she'd make comparisons in which most other men
fared badly. Richard had not only been handsome, but
humorous, bright, tender, and attentive. They had
shared simple enthusiasms: the lyrics of Cole Porter,
sailing, Edward Hopper's paintings. So desirable was
he, in fact, that she had been left asking herself whose
problem had really caused the breakup—his (as she'd
believed at the time) or her own? After two years in
which they had been perfectly compatible in bed, he
had begun suggesting that they put more spice into
their sex. He had wanted to bring in "toys"—as he
called them—a vibrator, ticklers, handcuffs. She had
uncomfortably tolerated it a few times, but then there
had been a furious argument, one winter weekend in
Vermont, when he had produced from his valise a new
purchase called *ben-wa* balls. She had barely listened
to the beginning of his lecture on the pleasurable uses
of the two small shiny metal spheres before letting fly
her resentment. For a long time afterward she felt
angry at how he had tried to pressure her.

"Don't be such a hung-up prude," he had said.
"This isn't going to hurt. It's all to make you feel
good."

But it didn't feel good. And calling her a prude, she
told him, was a form of dirty pool. She simply wasn't
ready to be the star of his pornographic fantasies—a
sex object accessorized like some damn sports car with
power steering. It had been all downhill after that,
right up to the breakup. Even the attempt at a recon-
ciliation several months later—despite the initial
warmth over dinner at Lutèce—hadn't gone further
than a single return to her bedroom. Richard called
occasionally since moving to Hartford to enter the top
echelons of an insurance company, and the conversa-
tions were always pleasant. But she could only mourn

the loss of intimacy between them—a casualty of the permissive modern age, the determined hunt for self-fulfillment without limit.

So it was difficult enough to build a relationship even when the man appeared to be—well, really *was*—wonderful. These days Carol no longer chided herself for making snap judgments about men; if there wasn't going to be at least a hint of chemistry right at the beginning, it was better not to take the first steps. If it meant being alone, then that was all right. She had wanted a career before she had wanted a man, and she wasn't sorry now even if she worried occasionally that she might be overdoing it—becoming "set in her ways," as another generation used to say about spinster ladies.

She would find someone, eventually, she was sure—someone as special and caring as Richard, but who would be the right man for the long run.

As the sky began to fade toward twilight, Carol rose from the couch and went out onto her small terrace. There were pots and windowboxes overflowing with impatiens and ivy, leaving room for only a metal café table and two chairs. In one corner Carol also cultivated a small tub of tomatoes. She had grown up in a house with a large yard, and though she felt no regret at leaving the suburbs for the city, she couldn't imagine living anywhere without access to some piece of outside space. The little terrace high above Second Avenue had been the deciding factor in renting the apartment.

She was plucking the few tomatoes that would be her last of the season when she heard the phone ring. Glancing at her hands, lightly coated with potting soil, she decided not to rush inside—the answering machine would take it. For half an hour she continued puttering with her plants, occasionally pausing to watch the sun go down over the city, then went inside, automatically throwing the bolt on the metal door. No intruder was likely to jump the three stories from the roof to the terrace, but you couldn't be too careful.

After washing up, Carol went to the phone machine on the night table in her bedroom and rewound the tape. The digital indicator showed there had been four calls since she'd gone out this morning. She hit the play button. The first beep was followed by the voice of her friend Margot Jenner with an invitation to drive up to her country house for Sunday lunch—"see the autumn foliage and all that."

Carol weighed the idea. It was nearly a two-hour drive to Rhinebeck, but being with Margot and her husband and kids provided a taste of family life that she always loved. She began to sort through her mail as the second caller came on, a man from the Canadian Film Board saying he was in town and wanted to meet with her about an animated version of *Tiger, Tiger,* her first book.

She had just opened the electric bill when the next message started. It was a woman's voice, the edge of extreme distress evident from her first quavering words:

"Oh, dear, Carol, this is no way to tell you . . . but even if you're not there . . . you'd still want to know, I'm sure, so you could try and . . . oh, God, how can I talk to this thing?"

The voice broke and for a moment only sobbing filled the tape. Carol ran a catalog of voices through her memory. Who was this? What tragedy could have struck?

A man's voice came on the tape, very somber, someone replacing the sobbing woman at the phone. "Carol, this is Ed Donaldson . . . Anne's father. We're calling all of Anne's friends to let them know her body has finally been found."

The muscles across Carol's abdomen suddenly constricted in a nervous spasm. She shuffled to the bed and sank down as the voice went on.

"There's a service here in Northport if you can make it. Eleven tomorrow morning, Church of the Ascension. Forgive us telling you this way, but there's so many people to call. . . . Well, I guess that's it."

The tape rolled on to the fourth message, the call Carol hadn't taken—a stockbroker she'd dated some months ago to say he'd been thinking of her, and was she free next Wednesday night?

Wednesday? The concept of future days to be spent in carefree pursuits suddenly seemed absurd. Only death seemed real right now.

. . . her body has been found . . .

Anne Donaldson had disappeared back in April. As long as no proof existed, no body, it had been possible to hope she was alive, a victim of amnesia or of some errant passion to escape a safe and familiar life and discover a new self. Carol had never honestly believed that, but now even those slim hopes were gone.

She went to the dresser and picked up a photograph of Anne and herself, side by side, smiling out from under their tasseled mortarboards at their high school graduation. A hundred memories of youth tumbled through Carol's mind all at once: sharing advice when they got their periods for the first time, later trading details about boyfriends, later talking about careers and later the love affairs—

But there would be no more "laters".

The tears flowed, finally, as the reality struck with renewed force. Anne was dead. No, not just dead: murdered. Carol wiped her tears and put the photograph back on the dresser. Tomorrow she would go to the funeral, and there would be a lot more crying. Right now she wanted to retreat from grief, and for her the best escape was in work. She had a real need for it, suddenly—to be inside her story, her world of fantasy.

Tonight, despite her grief, or perhaps because of it, she felt she would give birth to some truly wonderful monsters.

2 IT WAS AN INDIAN SUMMER DAY, warm for October—weather for a wedding, not a funeral. Smoothing down the skirt of her black linen suit, creased from sitting in church, Carol headed up the paved walk. At the door of the Donaldsons' white colonial-style house a group was trickling slowly inside. She guessed that Anne's parents must be standing there, receiving the visitors. The ceremonies at the church and the graveside had not provided an opportunity for the Donaldsons to accept condolences. Anne's mother, bent with grief and veiled in black, had entered the church leaning heavily on the arm of Anne's youngest brother, Skip. Mr. Donaldson had followed, eyes staring straight ahead, his posture artificially stiff, as though sworn not to be brought down by fate's worst blows.

From the moment Carol had seen them, she had felt there was something very different about this kind of funeral—the funeral for a murder victim. If an accident or a disease took the toll, the comforting generalities about life and death could soothe the pain. When Carol was only seven, her own mother had died after a long wasting bout with stomach cancer, and at the funeral there had been no end of people to assure her that "it was better this way." She had been to other funerals, too, of relatives who had died in serene old age and a boy she'd dated in college who died in the crash of his father's small private plane. In those cases you could feel a certain inevitability about the loss—

could say it was God's will, the ticking of the eternal clockwork.

But none of that made sense here. Anne's was a life snatched away by the deliberate act of another thinking being. It made no sense to say this was God's will—made God Himself seem senseless if He could allow some demented human to wantonly slaughter another.

Carol slowed on the sunny path. What could she say to the Donaldsons that wouldn't sound hollow and hackneyed? The nearer she got to the door, the more she was tempted to retreat, express her condolences in a letter. It would be immature, she knew, and yet a failure to grow up completely was a flaw she allowed herself. It was, in a sense, her stock-in-trade. If she preferred to shut out the world's horror, perhaps that gave a special poignancy to the fantasies she created in her books.

The knot of people around the door was shrinking.

After one more hesitation Carol continued forward. In the church and around the grave she had recognized a number of high school classmates she hadn't seen since graduation. It was a sad excuse for a reunion, yet likely to be the only way she would ever talk with old high school friends. And she felt there might be some special relief in sharing feelings about how Anne's murder had affected them.

As Carol stepped over the threshold, Mr. Donaldson greeted her. A gracious, handsome man with full iron-gray hair, he managed a slow smile.

"Carol . . . dear Carol," he murmured, his arms circling around her. "It helps to have you here."

She hugged him back and felt tears begin again. Her own father was not such a physically demonstrative man, and this was something she had always envied her friend.

"It's so awful," Carol said as Ed Donaldson released

her. "I keep wishing it could be a bad dream, and I'd just wake up."

"Wouldn't that be nice?" he said, and Carol realized her remark had been exactly the sort of vapid sentiment she had been afraid of spouting. He cut short the embarrassment for both of them by turning to his wife, who had just finished listening to the sympathetic platitudes of an elderly woman. "Sylvia, look who's here . . ."

Anne's mother took Carol's hand, then leaned closer and peered at her, mystified.

Sylvia Donaldson was still in shock, Carol realized.

"Carol Warren," she announced herself.

"Oh, goodness! Carol, of course. Isn't it terrible about my baby? The sweetest, loveliest person, wasn't she? How could anyone hurt such a sweet, such a . . . it's a dreadful world, isn't it? I'm not sure I even want to live in a world like this anymore. Maybe Anne's better off. Don't you think maybe she's better off?"

"I don't know about that, Mrs. Donaldson," Carol replied. "I only know I'm going to miss her terribly."

Carol hadn't noticed before the uniformed nurse standing to one side. But now the white-clad woman leaned over and asked Mrs. Donaldson if she felt like resting.

"No, I'm fine," Anne's mother said, then looked back to Carol. "It's nice to see you, dear," she added vacantly. "Please make yourself right at home. There's coffee and cake." She motioned loosely through a portal toward the living room, then turned to her husband, who was passing along the next visitor.

Carol moved ahead. There wasn't only one victim of a killing like this, she reflected. Sylvia Donaldson might someday regain something of her former self, but she would never really be the same. And who could say when, and at what cost, Ed Donaldson might finally exhaust the will that was holding him together?

Crossing the living room, Carol was struck by the

memory of a high school party here—an image of
Anne passing a plate of sandwiches, filling glasses with
Coke—but she was jolted out of the reflection by a
woman calling her name and making a beeline across
the room. In high school Debby Gahagen had been
among the prettiest and most popular girls, with a
brassy voice and blond hair that had combined to pass
for an enviable vivacity. Now she seemed a bit grace-
less.

"Carol," Debby gushed, "it's so great that you
came."

"Debby . . . what can you imagine I have to do that
would be more important than this? Anne was my oldest friend."

"Yeah. Mine, too."

In school, Carol remembered, Debby and Anne had
never been close.

"God," Debby went on, clutching at Carol's arm,
"after a thing like this, I don't know how anyone can
believe there shouldn't be capital punishment, do
you? How can anybody think it's enough, if they catch
this guy, just to lock him up? You don't let an animal
like this live. Not after what he's done to all these
women—"

Carol's glance had been wandering over other faces
in the room, but her attention was brought back to
Debby.

"Women?" Carol repeated. "Wasn't Anne by herself when—"

"Oh, she was alone when she was killed. They all
were." Debby Gahagen paused to study Carol's puzzled expression. "Haven't you been reading about
this? Last night's paper said whoever murdered Anne
might be a guy who's killed at least twenty or thirty
others."

"Thirty . . . ?" Carol mouthed, almost inaudibly.
Had she heard correctly?

"Maybe more. You really haven't followed this? The

papers have been writing about it for a more than a
year, on and off."

Carol shook her head, not only in answer, but in denial of the horror being described. It surprised her
only a little that she could have missed such a story.
She had the *Times* delivered, skimmed it front to back,
and listened to the radio while she worked. Yet she
often filtered out the constant stream of violent
events. It wasn't that she lived with blinders on, but
violence was only one thread in the broad fabric of city
living, and it was foolish to be obsessed by it. That,
of course, was the attitude she had been able to maintain until now—until one of her dearest friends had
been slain.

With evident pride in being better informed, Debby
Gahagen chattered on, filling in details she'd read in
the papers. Over the past eighteen months police had
begun to suspect that the deaths and disappearances
of a number of young women in several states—New
Jersey, Connecticut, New York, and Pennsylvania—
might be linked together, all committed by a so-called
serial killer. If there had been no superheated front-
page treatment of the story, it was apparently because
the police had little hard evidence to confirm their the-
ories.

"When Anne disappeared, the cops couldn't be sure
why," Debby explained. "But since they've found the
body, they're saying she fits the bill for one of this
guy's victims." Debby leaned closer to Carol, apparently pleased at being a giver of secrets. "She was
strangled *and* stabbed—that's something he does. The
body was in some woods, and she was naked, just
thrown out with not a damn thing on, and she'd
been—"

"Stop, please," Carol cut in, "I don't want to hear
any more."

The image of Anne had suddenly risen into her
mind, not as the nude, bloody corpse being described,

but the living picture of her, shrieking desperately and struggling with some shadowy attacker.

Debby Gahagen seemed surprised as Carol muttered, "Excuse me," then abruptly backed off.

She had an urge to run from the house, as if escaping could blank out the sadness. But she didn't want to make a scene. She glanced around for something to distract her from the awful shadows writhing in her brain, and her eyes settled on a man near the dining room table. He was in his mid-thirties, with a trim build, well-cut brown hair, and eyes a shade of blue bright enough to notice from across the room. As he leaned stiffly against a wall, not eating or drinking anything, he scanned restlessly from the new arrivals coming through the door to the groups of chatting friends and relatives. Recognizing that he was also ill at ease, Carol was tempted to approach him, make an alliance. But just then his roaming gaze came around to catch hers.

His slight smile hinted at shared distress, but it also felt like an invitation to an inappropriate adventure. She was here to mourn, not to enhance her social life. Denying herself the encounter almost as a sacrificial offering to Anne's memory, Carol looked away. As she turned, Ed Donaldson entered the room and came over. His wife had gone to lie down, he explained, had again been put under sedation.

"There are times I blame myself," he said.

"How can you . . . ?"

"When the police told us we'd have to"—he faltered for the barest instant—"make the identification, I let Sylvia go along. I tried to stop her, but she said it would be the last chance to see 'her baby' . . . and so I gave in." He went silent, staring at the floor. "Christ, they'd warned me how ugly it would be. But I just . . . never found a way to tell Sylvia exactly . . . make it clear just how bad—" Ed Donaldson cut himself short and for a long moment stared off into a vacant corner.

You mustn't blame yourself it's so terrible I loved her too

The platitudes marched through Carol's mind. But defeated by the certainty that none could help, she said nothing before Ed Donaldson turned back to her. "Well, somehow we'll deal with it," he said in his firm, heartbreakingly too-brave voice. "We will because we have to." He gave Carol's shoulder a gentle squeeze, then moved on across the room. Carol found herself wondering exactly what Ed Donaldson had failed to tell his wife about "just how bad" the experience of identifying their dead daughter would be.

Better not to know, she told herself, and decided she had stayed long enough. She was heading toward some old classmates to bid them good-bye when a voice spoke over her shoulder. "Can I get you a cup of coffee?"

Carol turned. It was the blue-eyed man who had been standing alone against the wall.

She hesitated, on the brink of telling him she was about to leave. "Thanks, but I'm keyed up enough today without coffee," she said, smiling to assure him she didn't mean to put him off.

"I can understand," he said. "Hell of a thing, isn't it? Did you know her well?"

"Best friends," Carol said. "And you?" Even as she asked the question, it struck her that he might well be a beau of Anne's.

"I didn't know her at all." He paused a second, frowning. "I'm working on the case. It's routine to cover the funeral when it's this kind of murder." He put out his hand. "Eric Gaines. I'm a detective with the New York City Police Department."

Carol introduced herself, gave him her hand, and for a moment they held each other in silent regard.

"Why is it routine," she asked, "for a policeman from New York to be out in Long Island?"

Eric Gaines smiled slightly. "That part isn't always

routine. But your friend disappeared in my jurisdiction."

"I see. But you said . . . when it's *this* kind of murder . . ."

He studied her as though trying to gauge the motive for her question—sincere interest or morbid curiosity. "The murderer in this case may be the kind of person who decides to show up here. And if he does, on the off chance we could spot him—"

"My God," Carol gasped, her glance sweeping over the crowd. "Do you think it's someone Anne knew?"

"No," the detective said, "it's not likely. But the killer still might put in an appearance. That's a wrinkle with some of these guys. They get a kick out of going to the church or the cemetery, watching the relatives cry. All part of their sick 'power trip.' "

Carol shuddered. "But surely someone like that couldn't come in here. A total stranger . . . he'd give himself away."

Gaines shrugged. "If it gave him enough of a charge he might still try—use a disguise, pose as a guy delivering flowers . . . or even as a cop."

At once Carol shied back. Gaines immediately dipped a hand inside his jacket, pulled out a worn leather folder, and showed her his badge. "I'm the real thing, don't worry." He slipped the folder back into his jacket. "But it doesn't hurt for people to be aware that anything's possible."

Carol thought of what Debby Gahagen had told her. "This case . . . is it really true that the same man may have killed thirty women?"

"Thirty, maybe forty. We don't really know."

"But that's got to be one of the worst murder cases in history. Why did I never hear about it until today?"

"Did you ever hear of the 'Green River Killer'?"

Carol shook her head.

"He's wanted in Seattle for the murder of thirty-seven women between 1982 and 1984. And thirty-seven is only the tally of victims whose remains were definitely identified. The cops out there have spent ten million bucks on the investigation and they've still got nothing. Maybe he's stopped, or maybe he's just moved on . . . come here." The detective took a deep breath and expelled it. "Hey, you don't really want to hear this. It's terrible stuff. Not what we—"

"But this man killed one of my best friends," Carol broke in. "It doesn't help to just . . . shut it out. The idea that these monsters can exist, and a lot of us don't even know."

"That's not so unusual," Gaines said mildly. "There's enough of these wackos around that they don't always make the headlines. Another body gets found, traced to a serial killer, and the story's buried on some inside page. The body may be someone who's been dead six months, a year . . . like your friend."

"Still . . . forty people," Carol said. "Half that number dies in a train crash and it's on the front page."

"Because it's a disaster—a lot of lives lost in one place at one time. The papers know how to focus on that. But take our investigation: it's been going on for almost two years—and we were late realizing we had a bunch of connected cases. When they get logged in over so much time, there's no momentum for the papers to build a big story." After a moment Gaines added, "And of course, we can't be sure there *is* a story. We've got so little real evidence, maybe we're cooking up something circumstantial—just to make ourselves feel better."

"I can't see how it makes you feel better to imagine there's a man roaming around who's already killed two or three dozen women . . . and you can't catch him."

Gaines gave her a rueful smile. "Perhaps it's a little better than thinking there may be seven or eight of these guys running around who've done five each."

He paused, then went on with forced brightness. "Okay, that's enough of this. When I walked over to you, my idea wasn't to give you bad dreams."

Then what was the idea? she might have asked. But she just didn't have the state of mind, in a situation like this, to allow herself to flirt. "I'll be all right," she said. "It was nice meeting you, Detective Gaines."

"Eric."

"Eric. I ought to be leaving now." She edged away.

There was a moment in which she thought he might ask if he could call, but instead he took out a business card, handed it to her, and said, "Nice meeting you, Carol. And please, let me know if you have any ideas about this case."

She decided then that he'd merely been on the job—subtly checking her out. If anything was possible, then perhaps this anonymous killer they were looking for was a woman. . . .

The talk with Gaines left Carol with the jitters. As she walked outside her eyes darted everywhere, searching for a suspiciously abandoned flower-delivery van, or a figure lurking behind a tree.

She couldn't help feeling safer when she got into her car, closed the door, and was driving away. So she was already passing a dark green station wagon parked at the end of Church Street when, from the corner of her eye, she noticed the man sitting behind the wheel. And only after turning and driving another block did it occur to her that she had seen him before—and would have recognized him sooner if he had been wearing the homburg.

Her heart began to pound, her hands tightened around the wheel, and her foot went to the brake. Yet she held back for another second. This, too, must be the aftermath of jitters aroused by the cop. She hadn't really gotten a good look at the driver's face; he could have been anyone, a local resident who'd just climbed into his car to go somewhere.

She drove another half block before deciding that it would bother her forever if she didn't check. She circled the block to come up behind the station wagon.

It was gone.

Probably just somebody who lived here, Carol told herself, or a repairman making a house call. Certainly not some maniac keeping a watch on the home of one of his victims.

Still, on the drive back to New York she kept checking her rearview mirror for the sight of a dark green station wagon with a driver who looked familiar. None appeared.

As soon as she got home, Carol tried writing a condolence note to the Donaldsons. Yet every phrase she set down seemed a belittlement of their pain and loss, so unnecessary and—she could only imagine—so cruel.

just how bad

The phrase uttered by Anne's father nagged at Carol the rest of the day, and into the evening. She went to sleep expecting to fulfill the police detective's prediction that he had given her nightmares.

She didn't have any, though. For that matter, she didn't dream at all.

3 SHE WAS ON THE ROAD early Saturday morning. Near the George Washington Bridge the traffic became a bumper-to-bumper caravan, but Carol was still glad to be headed out of the city. A party full of strangers might make her feel worse, of course, but she would try anything.

On the evening after the funeral her brother, Tommy, had been in Dallas on business, but he had called and quickly sensed how the day had devastated her. He assured her she could skip his housewarming. Instinctively, though, Carol knew that she ought to go. The new house had been finished only two months ago, and Tommy would want her there to share his pleasure.

Barely an hour into New Jersey, she pulled off the highway at Saddle River, a well-to-do suburb with substantial houses set on large tracts of pine forest. The driveways bore discreet wooden or metal signs, and some were blocked by wrought-iron gates with security cameras atop brick columns. The sign at the bottom of Tommy's driveway said only "Warren," no number. Carol turned in and drove to the top of a wooded hill, where a parking valet in a peaked cap waved the car to a stop. From the backseat she picked up the gift she'd brought, then got out in front of the house. It took her breath away. Though modern, it adapted Victorian touches—a planked gray exterior with white trim, soaring Palladian windows—and it was enormous.

At the front door she surrendered her coat to a uniformed attendant. "Mr. and Mrs. Warren are welcoming guests in the library," he said quietly, "down the hall to your right."

A rumble of conversation filtered toward Carol. She made her way to a high-ceilinged room where a fire roared in a deep flagstone fireplace. The crowd seemed mostly comprised of couples, and she felt a pang of unease. Was she to be a statistic, the only single person here? Entering, she saw Tommy and his wife, Jill, standing at the far end by the bar. As always, Carol was struck by how incredibly handsome her brother had become, with his thick auburn hair and sharply cut features. At one time his face had been softer, maybe too pretty, but in his thirties that had changed.

"Carrie! I'm so glad you came!" he called as he rushed over and gave her a hug.

"It's so beautiful out here. The house is really stunning."

"I wish Dad could have come," Tommy said.

"He would have loved it."

Softly Tommy said, "We can't let it go on like this much longer."

Carol nodded and a heavy silence fell between them—a symptom of their continuing failure to deal with the tragedy of their father.

"Are you okay?" Tommy asked at last. He kept his arm protectively around her shoulders. "You sounded sort of shaky on the phone."

"This thing with Anne," Carol said, "it's still hard for me."

"I know. I can't help thinking of when Mom died, the idea that you'll never talk to somebody again. And Anne . . . my God, she was so special."

Carol felt someone step up quickly behind her, but before she could turn, her eyes were covered by a man's hands.

"Guess who!" came the raspy voice.

She hadn't known he would be here today. "Must be . . . W. C. Fields," she said with a laugh.

"Gee, fooled you again."

Culley Nelson stepped around her. Her father's best friend was a big man with a broad barrel chest and a face permanently flushed red—by the blood of Scotland, he'd always joked, the kind that came in bottles.

"You look wonderful, sweetie," he said.

"How are you, Culley? It's so good to see you."

"I'm swell. And how about Tommy! Hell of a place he's got here, huh?"

Tommy smiled. "Hard work, Uncle Culley, that's all it takes. You and Dad always set a good example."

Culley Nelson worked at returning the smile. "I saw Pete yesterday. It's not good, kids. The time's comin' pretty soon when . . ." He paused, shook his head, then turned as a waiter passed carrying a tray of hors d'oeuvres. "Excuse me a sec', I think I'll feed my face."

As he moved away, Tommy whispered, "He's still the same, isn't he? Just a shy, happy guy."

Carol was about to express her agreement when Tommy's wife came toward them. Jill was slight but large-boned and had the round, sweet face of a madonna. When she and Tommy were married right after college, Jill had struck Carol as remarkably content in the role of dutiful wife, but this past spring she had gone back to school to pursue her own career. That, combined with Tommy's success, seemed to have given her a new self-confidence. Jill seemed less plain now, more poised. Her brunette hair was lightly tinted and done in a short feathered cut, a noticeable improvement over the girlish ponytail she had previously worn.

She took Carol's gift and unwrapped it. "Gorgeous!" she exclaimed, eyeing the set of antique Limoges demitasse cups. "Carol, you're an artist even when you buy presents. I wouldn't know where to find something this exquisite."

"Don't be silly," Carol said modestly.

"I hope you're feeling better," Jill said. "It must be awful for you . . . about Anne, I mean."

"Yes," Carol said flatly, eager to avoid a discussion of gruesome details.

Tommy led her off through the crowd and introduced her to his small corps of executives. Some of the men and their wives had brought copies of Carol's books to be signed for their children. She happily obliged and fielded questions about how she created her stories. Then Tommy escorted her out to a large buffet set up in the living room, where a waiter served cold filets of salmon and ratatouille.

"Nice, huh?" Tommy said.

"It certainly is," Carol replied as he led her to a chair. "And this house! I don't mean to be nosy, but are you sure you can afford this?"

"Who can afford anything?" Tommy answered with a laugh as he sat beside her.

"Seriously," Carol said.

"I wasn't going to tell you," Tommy answered, lowering his voice, "but it looks like we're taking Meditron public. Three years ago I never would have thought it could happen this fast. But if it does . . . good-bye to ever worrying about money. I'll have made a couple of my executives millionaires, too." He leaned close. "There's one of them here I want you to meet, his name's Frank Matheson. I think I told you about him, he's my right-hand man, and a great guy, too. We were at a Knicks game the other night, and he told me he's moving into the city, says it's too quiet out here for a single man, and I thought you—"

"Tommy . . . ," Carol interrupted in mild consternation.

"Okay, I don't mean to push, but I think you'd be much happier if you had somebody to share things with. You used to have more fun when you were with Richard. Since then . . . well, it seems to me you've been kind of drifting."

"I am not!" she said with a good-natured tinge to her protest. "I've been accomplishing a lot. Working, seeing friends—"

Tommy raised his hands in surrender. "Okay, maybe you don't need anybody new in your life. But Frank could use a friend in town. So maybe you can help him get settled—tell him about subways, that kind of thing."

Carol gave her brother an overdone frown.

"He's right over there by the piano," Tommy added, taking her silence as encouragement.

Carol peered across the room. "The one in the tweed jacket?"

The man caught Carol's eye, and Tommy waved him over. With his straw-blond hair and lanky, well-muscled body, Frank Matheson had an old-fashioned sort of good looks worn carelessly like a favorite old shirt. He was enormously attractive, Carol thought, and as Tommy introduced him he gave her the kind of smile that seemed to say everything was as right with the world as anyone could want.

"The teller of scary tales," he said. "I think your work is great."

"A glass of wine?" Tommy said. "I'll be right back."

Frank Matheson took a chair next to Carol.

"Have you actually read my books?" she asked. "They're for kids."

"Tommy gave me one," he said, *With the Night Creatures.* I'm very impressed, your drawings are so moving. Just looking at them, I felt a little like a kid again."

"How so?" Carol asked.

"I'd forgotten how frightening the world is when we're little, when everything seems so much bigger than we are. But seeing your drawings—that little boy lost in the woods and that giant squirrelly thing—I thought, gee, she's really good. You capture how it must feel to be a kid."

Tommy was right about Frank Matheson's charm, Carol thought. Most adults remarked more on her craftsmanship than on the emotional effect of the illustrations. And as she looked into his brown eyes, staring at the errant flecks of orange and green, Carol realized that for the first time in months she was feeling a strong flush of desire. It was the animal thing, she thought—when a man's face, his smell, the lilt of his voice, all combined to stir feelings over which you had no control.

"So you're moving to the city," she said.

"Yes, now that Tom's company is doing so well, I feel I can afford it."

"What do you do at Meditron?" Carol asked.

"Executive veep's the title. But you know, when a company starts up everybody's a cook and bottle-washer, filling in, doing overtime."

"I'm surprised you're moving away from all this bucolic beauty. I mean, with the long hours, why commute?"

Frank raised his eyebrows in a gesture of mock conspiracy. "Unless you're married, you could go bonkers out here. What these folks call nightlife . . ." He rolled his eyes. "Anyway, it's hard to meet people, and I worked for a while in Boston, so I miss sidewalks and being able to go out for a quart of milk at two in the morning."

She leaned toward him and felt the heat rise to her face. "Funny, isn't it," she said, "most people wouldn't call getting milk at two in the morning a big recommendation."

Tommy and Jill came over with Meditron's chief accountant and his wife, Alex and Estelle Gordon. Carol had met them before, and liked them both, yet regretted having her conversation with Frank interrupted.

Estelle Gordon, a vivacious, husky woman, planted herself on the adjoining chair and immediately reached for Carol's hand.

"Tommy told me about your friend, it's just horrible, you never imagine things like this happening to anyone you know."

Carol felt a flutter of despair. Was there no hope of avoiding the subject of Anne's death? Estelle Gordon probed for details, and while her questioning seemed at first inappropriate, her true concern soon made itself clear—her fears for herself and her college-age daughters, who both attended Barnard in the city.

"Where do these creatures come from?" she said. "What in hell is going on when a young woman can't walk on the streets without . . . oh, it's terrible."

"And inevitable," Frank said. "It's going to happen more and more."

"What do you mean?" Tommy asked.

"I saw a piece in the *Record* last week, an interview with a sociologist at Rutgers; he said that, morally speaking, we're not living in the same world we grew up in. A lot of it has to do with people not believing in anything, the rootlessness, so many people on the move, kids running away from home and living on the streets. So you get these serial murderers snatching people, and nobody notices. Like those two weirdos in California, the ones who were called the Hillside Strangler. A lot of the girls they picked up were runaways; nobody even noticed they were missing, let alone imagined they were cut up and lying in a ditch somewhere."

Carol listened as those around her lamented the decline of traditional values, but connecting these ideas to Anne's death struck her as insufficient to explain what had happened.

"Should we really be blaming society for these mon-

sters?" she asked. "Shouldn't people be held responsible for what they do?"

"Carol's right," Jill said forcefully. "I've been taking
abnormal psychology courses. These killers are psychopaths, they're men with sexual problems who have
to be violent toward women to get their kicks."

Tommy leaned forward. "It can't be that simple,
saying they have sexual problems. It's got to be something more. Some . . . I don't know, some force of
evil."

"You mean like the devil?" Estelle Gordon said.

"I don't believe in the devil," Tommy said, "but to
kill like that, again and again . . ."

The conversation drew the attention of several
other couples, who had gathered around, and Carol
noticed their looks of discomfort. "This has gotten a
little morbid," she said apologetically. "Let's change
the subject."

"I'll vote for that," Alex Gordon put in.

The conversation turned to housing costs in Saddle
River, and as unobtrusively as possible Carol slipped
away, moving over to the Steinway grand where a
hired pianist was playing Chopin. As Carol stood for
a moment, sipping wine, an image of Anne Donaldson's mother, her grief-stricken face, rose up in front
of her. Carol realized that the discovery of Anne's
body had been more unsettling than she could have
known, that somewhere in her mind a search had been
going on, as it always did in the face of death, for explanations, reasons. But there were none, no more
than for any death.

By the end of the afternoon Carol was able to take part
in the pleasure of idle chatter, the slightly drunken but
amusing jesting of Tommy's friends and business as-
sociates. She even managed to participate when
Tommy cajoled her into performing a duet with him

of a nonsense song they had liked as children, "Donkeys, Monkeys, Chickens in the Bed."

They had finished the last verse together when Carol turned to see Frank Matheson in a black bowler hat and a square paste-on mustache, waddling herkyjerky across the living room and swinging a cane from the tips of his fingers. He had metamorphosed into Charlie Chaplin, and the imitation was wonderful. With his loose linen pants lowered to his hips to seem baggy, and his face wearing the little-man-against-the-world gaze that Chaplin had so brilliantly used in *Modern Times*, Frank mimed trying to open a stuck door and falling flat on his face when it sprung at him. An invisible dog chased him and he tried to hit it with his cane as it tore at his legs. He got tangled on his cane and fell, stood up, then tripped on his hat and fell again.

Carol found herself laughing as hard as she had laughed in a long time; it acted like a tonic, lifting just a little the curtain of sadness that had surrounded her for days.

"Isn't he amazing?" Tommy said.

Carol agreed. "He's really a gifted mime."

Frank rested his arm on his cane and tipped his hat with an air of meek modesty, not stepping out of character for a moment and waiting while everyone applauded. Then he bowed again and came over to Carol.

"Madame approves?" He twitched the mustache Charlie-style.

Carol laughed. "Oh, very much," she said.

"I only do this when I want to win my Paulette Godard. So possibly you'll consider showing me the town when I move in, and perhaps allow me to squire you to a sumptuous meal."

Carol smiled as he bowed again, his arm thrown across his chest. No one had ever asked her for a date with quite such panache.

"Oh, yes," she said, letting her reserve slip. "I'd like that very much."

4 SHE WAS DEEP IN THE Cave of the Stone-Eating Blokes, quite hypnotized by the leader's green-and-purple-striped eyes, when a bell began clanging in the distance. Somewhere near the mouth of the cave, she thought, near the daylight.

Too far away to worry about.

Carol went on inking in the lines of a furry eyebrow, then heard a second ring and looked up at the phone next to her drawing table.

She waited for another ring, unable to remember whether or not she had turned on the answering machine. Wide-awake at five-thirty, she had made coffee and sat down to draw. Glancing around now at the clock-radio on the bookshelf behind her, she saw the digital numbers at 9:56. This was the first time the phone had rung today.

Carol picked up. As she brought the receiver to her ear, she leaned back and stretched the kinks out of her spine, causing her greeting to emerge in an unintended half-groan. " 'Lo . . ."

"Miss Warren?" It was a man's voice.

"Yes . . ."

The caller hesitated. "Is this a bad time to talk?"

It must have sounded as if he'd wakened her. "No, not at all. Who is this?"

"My name is Paul Miller. I'm—" He stopped short. "You sure I'm not interrupting anything? I need to talk to you for a while."

"About what?"

"It's a painful subject, I hate to bother you . . . it concerns Anne Donaldson. I'm one of the men working on the case."

"Oh, I see." Until this moment some part of her had still been in the cave, staying close to her fantasy. Now she was severed from it completely. "What can I do for you, Mr. Miller?"

"You were among Anne Donaldson's closest friends, weren't you? If we could talk, there might be something you remember that would provide a lead—something she said about her routine, who she was seeing, any special men in her life . . ."

"I certainly want to cooperate, but I don't see what I can tell you. Anne was killed by someone she *didn't* know—isn't that the police theory?"

"One theory, yes. But everything has to be covered. It might still be useful if I could sit down with you. Can we meet?"

In the policeman's sympathetic voice, Carol thought she heard something more than an awareness that he was treading in painful territory. A dedication to his work.

"All right," she answered. It was on the tip of her tongue to tell him he might as well come now, but at the last instant she changed her mind. After Anne's funeral she had found herself casting wary glances at strangers in the street, possessed by the notion that her friend's murderer was walking loose and could be anywhere—everywhere—around her. The feeling had waned, but Carol was far from tossing aside every precaution. Hadn't that other detective, Gaines, said that the sort of madman who'd killed Anne could even turn up in disguise at her funeral?

"Would it be all right," Carol asked, "if I came to your office?"

"I'm not going to be there today, but we don't have to talk in your home if that's what you're worried about."

Sensitive of him, she thought, then realized that of course it was a policeman's business to understand a woman's concerns about security.

He went right on. "Suppose I buy you lunch. There's a nice little spot called Sarabeth's Kitchen—on Madison, not too far from where you live."

"I know it." In fact, it was one of her favorite places, and she was impressed that the detective should suggest it.

"Can we meet there at one?" he asked.

It came to her again that absolutely nothing she could tell him would possibly be of any help. But how she could refuse? If there was the slightest chance . . .

"One o'clock," she echoed. "How will I—"

Miller anticipated the question. "I'll take a table by the window in the front room . . . and I'll be doing a crossword. I like puzzles to pass the time. See you later, Miss Warren."

After the call Carol picked up her coffee mug and went into the kitchen. A vague dissatisfaction grated on her, something so unfocused she wasn't sure if it was a subconsciously lurking problem with her work, or merely a minor stomach upset from nibbling on nothing but coffee cake since waking up.

Standing at the sink, rinsing her mug, the true source of concern broke through. Didn't policemen usually announce their rank, or connection to a particular precinct? But this man had given no identification beyond a name. Pegging him as a police detective had been her assumption.

. . . they get a kick from seeing the misery they created . . . might use a disguise . . . even a cop . . .

Carol ambled back to her drawing table. Gazing at the phone as if that might help her remember Paul Miller's words more accurately, she reran the conversation in her mind. He was working on the case . . . wanted to meet her.

Why did she find it troubling? Just nerves? Or intuition?

But what could happen in a public place?

Mindful that she often lost track of time while she worked, Carol went to the clock-radio and set the buzzer for twelve-thirty. Of course she must meet Paul Miller. He had said he was working on the case, that's all, had impressed her as being dedicated to solving her friend's murder.

She sat down again and picked up a sketching pencil as her mind rushed back into the cave.

Delayed by a call from her chatty editor just as she was leaving her apartment, Carol arrived at Sarabeth's Kitchen at almost fifteen minutes past the hour.

The sunny front area was furnished to create the ambience of a cozy English-style tearoom, with a counter at one side where jams, jellies, and baked goods were sold, and a few small wooden tables lined up across the window facing the street. The tables were all occupied by pairs of lunching women.

Again a notion stirred fleetingly that there was something not quite right about the phone call. Perhaps it had been a ruse to lure her from her house—?

Silly. No doubt it was as simple as all the front tables being taken when Miller arrived. She turned to the passageway that led back to a windowless rear dining room. As soon as she crossed the threshold, she saw a man at a table halfway into the room with a *Times* folded in front of him, a pencil in one hand. In the dim light she had to take another two steps toward the table before her eyes adjusted and his features—slightly masked behind a pair of half-lens reading glasses—became discernible.

Instantly her feet became rooted to the floor. For one more second she stared at him—and then the message came through to her brain. *Go . . . get out . . . get help. . . .*

But before she could move, he looked up, spotted her, and swept the spectacles from his face. Bunching the napkin from his lap, he rose to his feet and raised a hand. "Miss Warren," he hailed her past the intervening tables, "I'm Paul Miller."

The man from the bookstore. And now she knew that her imagination had played no tricks when she thought she'd seen him in a car near the Donaldsons' house. His interest was obviously not so much in following the thread of that case as in following *her*.

The murderer?

She couldn't conceive of it. If claiming her for a victim was his purpose, there had been opportunities enough without exposing himself this way. But then why? The feeling that he was dangerous lingered as she recalled the overture to this moment—that sly little scene where he'd bought a book, had her autograph it.

For several seconds they remained in a rigid tableau—she examining him fearfully, he waiting to see how she would react. At last he extended his arm and beckoned her forward. In a vagrant flash of memory Carol remembered being taken by her mother to visit a department store Santa—how terrified she had been, faced with the bulk of the huge man in red . . . until he had extended an arm and beckoned to her slowly as this man was doing now, a gesture that struck Carol as reassuring.

She glanced around, comforting herself that there were witnesses present, then moved toward him. Miller was tall enough to pull out her chair by bending across the table.

She sat, keeping her silence as he resumed his place. But the anger went on boiling up inside her. As soon as he was facing her across the table, she let him have it.

"Mr. Miller . . . frankly, your behavior has been unspeakable. If I had an ounce of sense, I probably wouldn't come anywhere near you."

A woman at the next table shifted her head for a sideways glance, making Carol aware of her own shrill tone. Leaning across the table she brought her voice down, though without sacrificing its sharp edge. "If you're really investigating Anne Donaldson's death, why didn't you tell me the first chance you had? And if that's not the truth, then you've got even more explaining to do. Unless you're pretty damn convincing, I'm going straight to the nearest phone to call the police."

Miller pursed his lips, his thick eyebrows went up, and he gave a slow rhythmic nod, as if accepting the chastisement. Then Carol saw a glint of bemusement creep into his eyes, and she felt he was observing her show of temper with detachment—an acting teacher approving a student performance of Lady Macbeth's mad scene. It should have infuriated Carol further . . . yet she felt disarmed. By treating her outburst as a performance, he implied that she couldn't possibly be afraid of *him*. And indeed Carol wondered whether she was as outraged as she'd tried to sound, or if she hadn't been laying it on a little thick.

"Well, aren't you going to defend yourself?" she asked.

He opened his hands. "What can I say? I'm not sure that the things you object to are defensible—by the usual polite standards. And you don't seem in any mood to accept a simple apology."

"I'm not," Carol declared. "What I want is a full explanation. Who are you? You're not a policeman."

"No," he said plainly.

"Well, then," she sputtered on, "what business have you—?"

"Ms. Warren," he broke in, "I agree with you. You have a right to a full explanation. But—as they say when hostile countries sit down to negotiate—do you think we might first try to 'normalize' relations . . . and order some lunch?" He motioned to the menu.

Trapped between feeling furious and disarmed, she was unable to answer and simply grabbed up the menu to hide her face behind it.

In the selection of tearoom staples on the menu—omelettes, waffles, salads—many were identified by names linked to childrens' stories or their enchanted world. "Baby Bear"—porridge with milk and honey; "Goldie Lox"—scrambled eggs with smoked salmon and cream cheese. Carol reflected on Miller's shrewdness in suggesting this place and decided it had been no coincidence. This man had a good sense of who she was, and had chosen a milieu to put her at ease.

How long had he been spying on her?

She lowered her menu to peer at him. With his reading glasses perched on his nose, he was concentrating on the menu. Her impression of several days ago struck her as not quite right; though at first glance he looked strangely severe, he was attractive in an unconventional way. His thick sandy hair had a frosting of white at the temples, but without the homburg he looked younger.

Miller caught her studying him. "Made up your mind?" he asked.

"Not quite," she said slowly, and looked back to the menu, though it wasn't the food she'd been talking about.

The waiter came over and she ordered the Fat and Fluffy French Toast while Miller asked for an Enchanted Garden Salad. She took a pot of tea, and he asked for a decaf.

As soon as the waiter collected the menus, Carol folded her hands and fixed her eyes on Miller. He watched the waiter walk away and then turned to her.

"So, how shall we do it?" he said amiably. "Question and answer? Or should I just take the ball and run with it?"

"Please," Carol said, "don't be flippant. This is my friend's murder we're talking about."

"Forgive me. It comes out of feeling so awkward, I suppose. But believe me, I was only trying to go about this in a way that would be easier on you—not to stir things up any more than I had to. I know it's put me in a bad light, and I'm sorry. Still, I'd like you to trust me."

Carol said nothing.

From Miller's grudging smile it was obvious that her message had come through loud and clear: her trust would have to be earned. Picking up his spectacles, he folded them back into his breast pocket. "I don't know if you're aware," he resumed, "that your friend's murder may have been related to a string of others, all committed by the same person. Perhaps as many as—"

"I do know that," Carol put in, the number of victims such an obscenity she couldn't bear to hear it repeated.

"One of the other victims," Miller went on quickly, "was a thirty-three-year-old woman from Oceanside, Long Island, who worked as a copywriter for an advertising firm here in the city. Her name was Helen Bonfarro. She disappeared about a year before your friend Anne—simply didn't come to work one day. Her parents reported her missing and worked through police channels for a while, but they felt the case wasn't being taken seriously enough. The woman had been romantically involved with a number of men her parents didn't approve of, so the police believed she'd simply gone off with one of them. That's when I came into it; I'm a private investigator. I went to work trying to locate Helen Bonfarro. Last spring she finally turned up in Connecticut. I didn't find her, though. A family on a picnic in a state park came across her naked body—or what was left of it—deep in the woods."

Carol shook her head sympathetically. From the hoarse tone that had crept into Miller's voice, she could tell the case had become more to him than merely a job.

"I'm still with it," he went on, "because there's still a question of who killed Helen Bonfarro. Was it a murder committed by someone she knew . . . or is she a random victim of the same man who murdered your friend? Trying to answer that question leads to all the cases that might be related." He fell silent, as though waiting for confirmation that she had followed his explanation.

"What you're telling me," Carol said, "is that you're not actually working on the Donaldson case."

"Not exclusively," Miller said. "But I'm very concerned with it—in fact, with every murder that might be a link. Understanding any one of these killings might shed light on another. Studying similarities could help determine if the Bonfarro case should be consigned to the same investigation as Anne Donaldson's."

The waiter arrived. As the tea and coffee were set down, Carol looked across the table and weighed what she'd heard. An oversight occurred to her, a demand she should have made earlier.

"Mr. Miller," she said, "I believe I'm correct that private detectives need to be licensed. Can I see your license?"

He blinked at her, as though caught off guard. Carol was certain he was working to concoct an excuse for being unable to oblige her request. With an air of forbearance, however, he pulled a wallet from his jacket. Flipping it open, he delved under a flap and came up with a small laminated card. It appeared to certify that one Paul D. Miller had been licensed as a private investigator by the State of New York.

As she handed it back, Miller said, "You really shouldn't be won over by that. Mandatory it may be, but carrying it puts me in a dubious brotherhood that includes various mafiosi, strong-arm thugs, and other forms of undesirable streetlife."

She ignored the attempt to deprecate her caution and said coolly, "Now you can explain why you weren't straight with me. Following me around, pretending to buy a book—"

"I didn't pretend," Miller corrected. "I paid for it and took it home."

"Don't fence with me, Mr. Miller," Carol snapped.

Miller bowed his head. Carol couldn't tell if he was indeed chastened—or merely aping a meek schoolboy to belittle her anger.

"I bought the book and had you sign it," he said, lifting his head again, "because it was an easy way to obtain a sample of your handwriting."

Carol stared at him dumbfounded. A sample . . . ? Did he mean he had been collecting evidence? "Good god," she said, shocked, "why would you think that was necessary?"

"Desirable," he said, "not necessary. The police let me see the contents of a purse that was found with Anne Donaldson's body. Inside were a couple of sheets from what must have been a longer letter, the signature page missing. The letter was undated, and much the worse for wear since the purse had been exposed to the elements for several months. It could have been something she'd carried around for a long time, or received the day she disappeared. The police couldn't tell. But the letter was filled with stuff about ending a relationship. I'll spare you the details, but it was clearly from a woman who didn't want to go along with Anne's desire for . . . a deeper friendship. Hard to say where such friction might have led."

"That's absurd," Carol burst out. It was ridiculous—the idea that she could have killed Anne to escape an unwanted lesbian affair.

Miller shrugged. "I told you, Miss Warren, that my

first impulse was to go about this in a way that spared us both."

"And what have you found out now, Mr. Miller?" she asked sharply. "Have you discovered that I killed Anne?"

"Of course I haven't."

Her angry tone heightened. "Because my handwriting didn't match the letter?"

He regarded her with weary tolerance. "Do you think every possibility shouldn't be checked out? Is that the way you'd like an investigation of your friend's murder to be handled? Maybe the police are willing to skip over possible evidence, draw their own dainty conclusions, but I'll be damned if I am."

Carol looked away. With grief and anger colliding inside her, she felt on the verge of tears. She put her hands up and rubbed at her eyes with her fingertips. "It's hard to behave well in a situation like this, isn't it?" she asked. "Whether you're a detective or a suspect."

Miller smiled slightly. "That's why I sometimes take the easy way out."

The waiter returned with their food and they both began to eat. Normalizing relations, Carol mused.

"It sounds as though you've become just as involved in Anne's case as in the first one," she said. "Are the Donaldsons paying you, too?"

He shook his head and swallowed his food. "I thought I'd cleared that up. The Bonfarro and Donaldson murders may be linked. Solving one could solve the other."

"Wouldn't that be true of any case that might be traced to this one killer?"

"Yes."

"The police said there might be as many as forty related cases," she said. "Are you looking into all of them?"

He swallowed a piece of tomato and went after a

disk of cucumber. "There have been, over the past few years, a total of twenty-nine women whose bodies have been recovered, and who—from a certain amount of forensic evidence—can almost positively be categorized as victims of the same killer. Beyond that, we can only speculate, including in the count any missing women from the areas where other killings have occurred." He looked up. "But yes, I'm covering as much ground as I can."

His hazel eyes held hers in a burning gaze, and Carol realized that the pursuit of an answer had become much more than a paid assignment. It didn't seem necessary to ask some of the other questions that troubled her. Why had he been watching Anne's house? For the same reason as Detective Gaines, she assumed—to survey the mourners, watch for anyone suspicious.

But one question still hadn't been satisfactorily answered. "Why did you want to see me today?" Carol asked, her tone deliberately suspicious.

Miller appeared surprised by the question. "I told you, didn't I? I want your ideas on the case. Anything you can think of that might help."

"But I don't think there could be anything."

He pushed his salad bowl aside and leaned in closer to the table. "Look, you grew up with this woman. To me she's just . . . well, you do get to know the victims in a way when you study them enough, but never like the people who knew them when they were alive— family, close friends, lovers."

Carol was stumped. It still struck her as hopelessly optimistic to imagine she held any key. "I don't have any clues to what happened. I accept what the police say—that Annie was a random victim."

"Do you know anyone she was seriously involved with? Anyone at the time of her death?"

"No one, not as far as I know. But I doubt she confided everything to me. Our lives had gone in separate directions. We met occasionally, had dinner in town. But the last time was several months before she disappeared."

"And she didn't mention any . . . attachments?"

Carol thought back to the last time she'd seen Anne. Where had they gone? Hard to pin it down now. Was it the time they'd pulled strings to get tickets for *Cats*, and then found themselves so horrendously bored they'd walked out and gone for a Mexican dinner? Even then, unexpectedly smashed on margaritas, Anne hadn't complained about any men. Or women.

Carol's attention came back to Miller. "No, she didn't mention anyone special. But why are you harping on this, Mr. Miller? Aren't you trying to find a serial killer—someone who picks his victims haphazardly?"

"Yes. I'm also trying to ascertain who his victims are—or aren't. It could be that Anne Donaldson doesn't belong in the group, that she was the sole victim of a crime of passion by someone she knew."

Carol raked once more through her faint memories. "I'm sorry. I can't remember anything significant."

Miller's eyes remained on her for another moment. Then a smile broke over his face, almost incongruously sunny when compared with the grim intensity that had preceded it. "Well . . . that's it, I guess. It was a long shot, but I had to give it a try. There's so little evidence." He signaled for the bill, throwing his hand up in an overblown gesture that couldn't fail to catch the waiter's eye.

"You'd think," Carol said, "that anyone who committed thirty or forty murders would leave a trail a mile wide."

"It should work that way, but there seems to be a certain safety in numbers. You're talking about people who commit murder as efficiently as . . . a carpenter building a bookshelf. They get their materials, take their measurements, and do their job. And the more they do it, the better they get . . . until even the smallest little rough spots are smoothed out."

Carol shuddered at the description. "You make it sound as if this one might never be caught."

"Did I?" The check had been brought to Miller. He stared down at it intently. Carol thought he was going over the addition until he spoke. "No, he'll be caught."

Miller took his wallet from inside his jacket, counted out several bills into a neat stack, and laid them at the center of the table. A very precise man, Carol thought as she watched, very careful about the way he did things.

And then she heard him say it again, very softly, his eyes still aimed down as if he were looking through the table to something beyond, even far below the surface of the earth: "He will be caught."

Miller stood quickly, went to the passageway where his overcoat and hat hung on a rack. He slipped into his coat, then fitted the homburg to his head, adjusting it to a very slight angle. All without acknowledging Carol, as if he were already embarked on some solo mission. At last, however, he turned to her and made a small courtly sweep of his hand, inviting her to precede him out.

In the street he said, "Can I take you anywhere? I have a car." He pointed across the avenue. By a meter stood the green station wagon—the one Carol had spotted near the Donaldsons.

She didn't doubt the things Miller had told her, didn't even doubt that he was deeply involved in the hunt for a serial murderer. And yet she also felt that something about Mr. Paul Miller deserved her suspicion.

"Thanks, but no," she said. "I have an errand to do right around the corner."

He smiled in a way that seemed to accept she was merely making a polite excuse. "It was nice of you to meet me," he said. Then he tipped his hat slightly and strode away.

A careful man, Carol thought again, noting that he went to the corner to cross the street—even though the traffic was sparse and he could have cut across directly. The kind of man who took no chances. Not so very different, she imagined, from the kind of man he had described as capable of getting away with murder after murder.

But then, of course, the same qualities were undoubtedly an asset in the hunt.

5 IT WAS EARLY EVENING, as she walked up
Second Avenue to the dry cleaner, when Carol
saw ahead of her a man in an overcoat with broad
shoulders and a slow, purposeful gait. For a moment
she thought it was Paul Miller. But after he stopped
at the window of a drugstore she caught sight of his
face in the dim twilight. He looked nothing at all like
the man she had met for lunch.

Yet the mere thought of Miller set off a queasiness
in her. Why had she sat there so compliantly, revealing
personal feelings about Anne to a man she had never
met before? Miller had been so adept at soothing her.
Too adept, perhaps.

Carol began to feel foolish . . . worse than foolish.
She thought back over her conversation with him. He
had mentioned another murdered woman, a family in
Oceanside, Long Island, with an Italian name . . . Bonfarro.

Arriving home after her walk, Carol headed for the
living room phone and dialed Long Island information. There was a John Bonfarro in Oceanside, on
Knight Street. Carol hesitated, mulling the possibility
that this was an irrational thing to do. Then she made
the call, punching the number quickly before she
changed her mind.

It rang eleven or twelve times, and Carol was about
to give up when a woman answered with a breathless
"Hello."

"Mrs. Bonfarro?"

"Yes?"

"I'm terribly sorry to bother you, but I'm calling to . . . this is hard to explain . . ."

The voice on the other end had a gruff, harried quality. "Look, if you're selling something, can you call back later? I'm doing a laundry."

"Please, Mrs. Bonfarro, this will only take a minute."

"All right, if that's all."

"My name's Carol Warren, and I had a friend who lived out near you, Anne Donaldson."

Carol heard a sharp intake of breath. "What do you want?" the woman asked, her tone growing clipped, guarded.

"My friend Anne—"

"I saw about it in the paper. What's that got to do with me?"

Carol pushed ahead. "I'm really sorry to bring this up, but apparently the death of your daughter—"

"Listen here, miss, what are you—some ghoul, calling up to make me crazy with my memories? I don't have nothing to say about that, it's all done now. I'm gonna be hanging up—"

"Wait," Carol pleaded, "can't you give me a minute? The private detective you hired, Paul Miller, he told me that my friend Anne's death and the death of your daughter might be connected."

There was a long pause. "Listen," the woman said, her voice quavering, "we never hired a private detective. We don't know anybody named Miller, and I don't know you either. So I'm getting off now, and don't you call again or you'll make me get hold of the police."

The connection was abruptly broken.

Carol hung up and stood by the phone as she mulled her own stupidity. To have accepted Paul Miller so easily . . .

If the Bonfarro family had not hired him, who was he? Why had he been stalking her?

She went to her drawing board, thumbed through the papers piled in the corner, and found the card she'd taken from the policeman at Anne's funeral—Eric Gaines. It gave his number at the 112th precinct in Queens. Carol picked up the phone.

"One-one-two, Panetta," came the voice after she had dialed.

Carol asked for Eric Gaines.

"Detective Gaines is out. If you leave your name and number, I'll tell him when he comes in."

"Is there a way to get in touch with him? This is . . . kind of an emergency."

"*Kind* of an emergency?" the voice repeated a bit tiredly.

"I just need to talk to him. Could you tell him Carol Warren called—tell him we met at Anne Donaldson's funeral?"

Carol heard a shuffling of papers. "Donaldson . . . that the girl from Northport?"

"Yes," Carol said.

"Wait a sec, Miss Warren."

The police officer returned in a minute. "Miss Warren, do you have a car?"

Carol said she did and was told that Detective Gaines would be able to meet her at an address in Brooklyn if she could get there within the next few hours.

"Brooklyn? I don't understand."

"He's on a case, Miss Warren. And he expects to be there most of the evening. But he said he'd like to see you if you could come down there to talk to him."

Carol quickly wrote down the directions.

On Court Street in Brooklyn she nearly missed the low building she had been told to look for, the offices of Brooklyn Federated Gas. In this neighborhood of mom-and-pop corner stores and chic boutiques, the company's headquarters was all but camouflaged behind a row of leafy elms. If not for the red-tipped yellow flame painted on the glass doors, Carol would have driven past it.

In the tiled lobby a security guard took her name, then directed her to the third floor. When the elevator doors opened, Carol stepped into a huge fluorescent-lit room—the company's credit division, according to a sign mounted on a pole. The air was stuffy and overheated, and on rows of folding chairs dozens of people sat reading newspapers and quietly chatting—employees of the company, Carol assumed. Gathered around a table in a corner were several uniformed policemen. She approached and asked where she could find Eric Gaines.

"He's seeing everyone in order, miss," one of them replied. "If you'll just wait till they call your name . . ."

When Carol explained that she had come at Gaines's invitation, the oldest of the policemen politely asked her to wait while he went looking for the detective.

Carol sat in one of the folding chairs, and in a moment she saw Eric Gaines coming toward her from the far side of the room. He had taken off his suit jacket and loosened his tie, and Carol couldn't help noticing his gun in its shoulder holster, stark against the white of his shirt. With his grim expression and rumpled hair he had a weary look about him.

"Miss Warren, hi." He shook her hand. "Sorry to keep you waiting."

"I shouldn't have bothered you, I know—"

"The precinct said something about an emergency."

"Maybe I'm overreacting, but . . ." Carol looked around, aware that people were staring at her.

Gaines noticed it, too. "Come on in here," he said,

and led her into one of several windowless cubicles along a wall.

Inside were a wooden desk and two chairs. The air had a musty smell, like a closet that hadn't been cleaned in years.

"We've taken this place over for the night," Eric said. "Can I get you some coffee? A Coke?"

"No, thank you."

"You sure got here in a hurry. What's the emergency?"

Carol reported Paul Miller's phone call and her meeting with him at Sarabeth's Kitchen, and her certainty that he had been lurking on the street near the Donaldsons' house.

"Did you actually see him at the funeral?" Eric asked.

"There was a man behind the wheel of a green station wagon," Carol said, "and Miller had one when I met him for lunch. But at the time I wasn't sure. Maybe I should have come back to the house to tell you."

"Hey, it's all right," Eric assured her, "I'm not blaming you, you had other things on your mind. But go on, tell me what happened after he called."

She recounted Miller's claim to having been hired by the family of Helen Bonfarro. "But when I called the girl's mother, she'd never heard of Miller. I'm just so damn scared now. I told him all about myself, and he's obviously been tracking me."

Eric reached over and gently touched her hand. "Hey, it'll be fine, Carol . . . I mean, Miss Warren."

"It's all right, you can call me Carol."

Eric smiled briefly, pulled a stenographic notebook from his back pocket, and then urged her to run through her concerns again, dredge her memory for anything specific. Anything unusual about his looks, manner, clothes?

The only thing that stuck in Carol's mind was the homburg.

"It didn't seem appropriate somehow," she said. "When he took it off, he looked like a different kind of person . . . as if it wasn't his normal choice of clothes."

And then she thought of one other thing—the anonymous letter found in Anne's purse, and Miller's explanation that he had wanted a sample of Carol's handwriting.

"A letter?" Eric said curiously. "I know that case upside down and sideways, and there was no letter in Anne Donaldson's purse."

"Oh, Jesus, he made that up, too."

Eric tapped his pencil on his notebook. "Carol, I don't know how much I can do about this now. His real name might not even be Miller. I'll run a check on it and see what I can turn up." He closed the notebook. "In the meantime, if you hear from this man again, don't waste any time calling me at the precinct. And if the guy actually tries to get near you, just stall him long enough for me to get there. Okay?"

"Okay," Carol said. The detective's assurances made her feel better, and she smiled at him in appreciation.

There was a knock on the edge of the partition, and a blond man, also in a shirt and tie, poked his head into the cubicle.

Gaines turned to him. "Yeah?"

"Sorry to butt in, Lieutenant, but we're finished with the late-shift people. Unless you want to do them again."

Eric dabbed at his cheek with his shirtsleeve. "Did we get a list of times for all of them?"

"Yeah, for each one."

"But did you line up the times so we know who came in right before she disappeared and right after?"

The other detective looked embarrassed. "Not yet, no."

"Christ," Eric said, annoyed. "Before you let anyone go home, I want to see each person who came or left within ten minutes of when she walked out that door—before *and* after she walked out." Eric grimaced. "Did you get a list of the people on the early shift who smoke?"

"No, sir, why?"

"Because you can't smoke in this building, Jerry, it's against the law. So somebody might've been out in that lot taking a smoke break when the guy pulled his car in. And if we know who the smokers are, we can call 'em all in here tonight instead of starting from scratch in the morning."

"I'll get right on it," the other detective said.

"Yeah, okay," Eric said frustratedly. "Do that." He turned back to Carol. "We have more than a hundred interviews to do tonight. I guess you heard why."

"A woman has disappeared," Carol said. "Is it the same as . . . ?"

Eric shrugged. "Could be," he replied. "And we may actually be on to something. Stick to it long enough, you finally get a small break. Tonight I think we got one."

The missing woman, Eric explained, was a young junior executive who had left her office late, on her way to a meeting in Manhattan. A second woman, who worked on the night shift answering emergency service calls, had arrived for work at the same time that the executive was leaving.

"Behind this building there's a parking lot. Our witness thinks she saw the victim—I mean the woman who's missing—being helped into a car by a man on crutches."

"So this man is disabled?" Carol asked.

"Not quite." Eric paused. "Carol, I want to confide in you, but you've got to understand how delicate this

is. If any of what I tell you shows up in the papers or
on the six o'clock news, it'd destroy our ability to use
it as evidence, or to weed out the crazies who confess
to any crime, or—"

"I understand," Carol broke in.

He studied her another moment, then went on.
"With all these disappearances, one thing has
stumped us. Why did these women go willingly with
a man they didn't know? A lot of them were profes-
sionals—savvy, high-achiever types in their thirties.
Like your friend Anne Donaldson. You'd expect them
to be smart, not the kind to get lured easily into a trap.
Yet we've never had a single witness report a struggle,
or even a scream. So how is this killer getting to them?
Of course we figured he had a knack, a good line, the
gift of gab, maybe a prize-winning smile—"

"But the crutches would clinch it," Carol blurted as
comprehension broke through.

"Bingo. What could make a guy easier to trust?
What's your first impulse when you see a guy on
crutches? You want to help. Until tonight we didn't
know anything about this guy, we didn't have a single
eyewitness, but now we know how our killer can catch
his victims off guard."

Carol was seized by the realization that she conformed to the general profile of the victims Eric had
described—attractive career women in their thirties.
And she, too, was perhaps overly trusting, could fall
for a good line, as she had for Paul Miller's. Her brow
furrowed as she looked up at the detective.

"I have a hunch I'm upsetting you," Eric said, "and
you came out here to get over being upset." He stood.
"What I'd like to do is take you out for a sandwich and
talk about something else. But I can't. If you don't
mind, though, I'd like to call you."

The concern was obviously more than professional.
Carol was flattered and said she wouldn't mind at all
if he called.

He walked her to the elevator and pushed the call button. "Remember: if you hear from this guy, let me know, don't wait a minute." He reached into his pocket. "Here's my card."

Carol smiled. "You gave me one, I have it at home."

"Take another to keep with you, in your purse."

The elevator doors opened, and Carol got in. As the doors closed, she heard Eric call out a tired good-night. It hit her then that he had been exactly right about his effect on her. She had come here tonight because she was upset and frightened. She had wanted to be comforted. But instead she was leaving more frightened than ever.

6 "LOOK AT THAT SKYLINE," Frank Matheson said. "Is there a more exciting place on earth than this city?"

They were on the ferry crossing back toward Manhattan after touring the Statue of Liberty, Frank's idea of a way to spend Sunday afternoon, their first date. "Let's be tourists for a day," he had said when he called Friday, and the suggestion had charmed Carol at once. In fact, it was part of Frank's appeal in general, she was discovering, a somewhat naive enthusiasm for things that many people might dismiss as corny or commonplace.

Carol turned to look out over the rail at the spectacular view of skyscrapers on the city's southern tip. "It is magnificent," she said, and groped unsuccessfully for something more. She had been poor company today, she knew, but it was hard to match Frank's brio while she was so preoccupied.

All through the afternoon, while Frank had talked about the newfound pleasures of living in a city again, and tried to entertain her with stories of his boyhood in Fall River, Massachusetts—"you know," he had said, "the place where Lizzie Borden took an ax"—Carol's attention had constantly drifted away to search the lines waiting at the statue and to check the faces of people on the ferry.

"Where would you like to have dinner?" Frank asked. "I was thinking we might try Windows on the World."

"Dinner?" she answered distractedly. She had lapsed into gazing through a window at the ferry's inner cabin, where the people who wanted to stay out of the wind sat on long benches. Crusted with dried salt from the sea spray, the window offered only a murky view. At the end of one row, was there a man in a brimmed hat?

"Oh, I see," Frank said, making his own interpretation of her lackluster response. "You'd rather not stretch this out any more."

"No, I'd love to have dinner with you."

He hesitated. "Are you sure? Don't do it just to be polite—because I'm Tom's friend. You gave it a shot, Carol, I appreciate that, but sometimes these things just don't work out."

It took another moment before she focused on him completely and realized the source of the misunderstanding. "I'm sorry, Frank," she said, "I know I haven't been much fun. But it's not because of you. I liked the outing, and you've been lovely."

He shrugged and gave a slight smile, a winning show of modesty. "I don't get it, then. I was sure you were bored stiff."

"No, it isn't that." Carol paused. "I've been wondering all day," she said with a small self-deprecating laugh, "if there hasn't been someone following me."

"Following you? But why . . . ?"

In her relief at having Frank to confide in, it all poured out nonstop—the man who had been stalking her, the funeral, the meeting at Sarabeth's.

"It's been kind of . . . nerve-racking," she said, "and when I spoke to the police, and learned that there wasn't any note in Anne's purse—that this man Miller had made it all up—it really tipped me over the edge."

Frank studied her with obvious concern. "I wish you'd explained this earlier, Carol."

"I guess I've been trying not to admit how much it's been bothering me."

"That's only natural," Frank said. "What did the police say about this guy?"

"To call them if he shows up again."

"That's all?" Frank said.

"This police detective I talked with—he's working on cases like . . . like what happened to Anne—he didn't see what else he could do unless I was bothered again."

Frank nodded. "Tell me once more about the bookstore. It does sound spooky. You said he struck you as strange right away."

Carol told him about her first impression of Miller, her feeling of being examined, but then Frank interrupted.

"When you met him for lunch," he asked, "did he show you any credentials?"

Carol felt the questioning had gone on too long. She needed Frank's moral support, not a show of impatience with the way she had handled the situation. "Look, if he bothers me again, I'll just call the police and they'll take care of it." The ferry bumped into its slip. "Let's go and have a nice dinner somewhere."

Frank reached over and touched her hand. "Sure, whatever you say."

Without reservations they were turned away from Windows on the World, but they walked the streets of Tribeca and found a nice Italian restaurant. Carol resolved to keep thoughts of Paul Miller at bay, and at last the conversation between her and Frank began to flow easily. He spoke of the cooperative apartment he'd bought and his planned renovations; she revealed her dream of illustrating Grimms' fairy tales in an entire new series of books. By the time they were in a cab heading back to her apartment, she felt she was lucky to have met Frank and was certain she wanted to see him again.

*　　*　　*

"I had a wonderful day," she said warmly when they reached her lobby.

"Me, too," Frank said, heading for the elevator.

Carol hesitated. She thought of asking him up but imagined he might take the invitation the wrong way. "If you don't mind, I'm feeling a little worn out."

Frank seemed taken aback. "What, no nightcap?" he asked, his hands turned up in mock supplication. "You'd send a man into the cold without a shot of spirits to protect him?"

"It's been a long day, Frank, and I'm a little edgy, and—"

Frank dropped his jovial pose. "I was only suggesting a drink. I wasn't planning on . . . trying to take advantage of a lady." He put his arms around her waist. "When am I going to see you again?"

"Soon, I hope." She gave him a brief kiss. When his arms remained at her waist, she eased back, delicately letting him know that it was as far as she was prepared to go tonight.

In the elevator she leaned against the brass handrail, exhausted. Maybe she should have invited Frank up for a nightcap. The truth was that she found him attractive and had sent signals saying so.

Stepping into her dark apartment, she wondered about herself. She remembered how she had felt in the months after breaking up with Richard. Friends and lovers came and went, she told people, that was the nature of these things. She would announce to anyone that she cherished her "privacy," when the real word, she knew, was "loneliness."

So maybe, she thought, she had been too standoffish with Frank. Not all men were going to make the demands that Richard had—reveal themselves, behind the caring facade, as wearing the horns of a satyr.

The next time she was with Frank, she resolved, she would try to be more open to all the possibilities.

7 UNNERVED BY A SILENCE that had already lasted several minutes, Carol rose from the chair opposite Binny Madison's desk. She paced to the window and gazed down for a second at the streetscape twenty-six stories below, then turned back to watch her editor, who stood slowly turning the large folio cards on which Carol had presented the illustrations for her new book. Binny Madison was a sixtyish gamine woman with kohl-rimmed eyes and a bowl-cut wig so intensely black it actually reflected the light from the window like a dark mirror. She was given to wearing oversize shifts and long necklaces of pottery beads. But if Binny's sense of personal style was questionable, Carol knew that her editorial judgment was nearly infallible.

Finally she heard Binny emit a low ruminative purr, a sound that always meant the editor was postponing some negative comment.

"All right," Carol burst out, "so you don't like them."

Binny plopped down into her large swivel chair, her beads clattering against the desk. "I didn't say I didn't like them. They're beautifully executed as always, dear, the whole sequence of Dana in the underground city is so imaginative and the coloring is lovely—"

"And what's wrong?" Carol said.

Holding up one of the pages so that it was caught by the sun beaming through the window, Binny Madison examined it as a doctor might peer at an X ray to make a harsh diagnosis.

"This is only the most subjective reaction, you understand," she offered at last in an apologetic tone, "but there's a kind of morbid air that hangs over some of these drawings. I mean, here, where Dana is grabbed up and flown away by these huge winged creatures—what do you call them?"

"The Flybyes," Carol said, unable to keep the testiness out of her tone. It was a weakness, she knew, but she often had trouble dealing with criticism.

"Mmm, a nice name," Binny chirped. "But where you show them gripping Dana, there's such careful detail of the talons, and the way they're digging into the child's skin . . . well, it just looks unnecessarily painful."

"Oh, for God's sake, Binny. Not you—you're not going to hit me with that nonsense we get from the child psychologists about my books being too disturbing. My work is a lot less terrifying than the Brothers Grimm, and there's a release for kids in being able to see their nightmares fleshed out as fantasy."

Binny continued shuffling through the stack of matte cards to which the drawings were taped. "This one," she sighed, "where Dana's in the cave with those Bloke creatures. Look at these details around the walls. Skeletons of animals . . . some of the bones even have carrion clinging to them."

"What did a caveman's home look like, Binny? Wall-to-wall carpet?"

Binny tossed the card down. "This isn't your best, dear. Why defend it?"

"Maybe it's just too hard to do my best all the time."

Binny eyed Carol for a moment, then waggled one of her bony fingers commandingly in the direction of the chair opposite hers. "Now, what's bothering you, dear?"

It was on Carol's tongue to dismiss the question as

absurd, when she realized the truth. She sat down. "A friend of mine was murdered, her body was found only last week. Those two drawings you picked out . . . I did both of them after learning about it."

"Ah," Binny said softly. "I'm sorry. But I can certainly understand how that works its way in . . . a loss of faith in the world as a decent place."

"I didn't understand it until this second," Carol said. Hadn't understood either, she realized, that her negative perspective wasn't merely tied to one murder, but to thirty or forty, all of young career women not so different from her.

Binny gave her a gentle smile. "Would you like to talk about it?"

Carol shook her head. "I'm okay."

"So . . . you think these can be reworked a little?" Binny closed the folio and pushed it across her desk.

Carol smiled. "Sure."

"On your way then, pumpkin."

Carol rose. The meeting had been much briefer than usual. "Give me a few more days," she said, tying the string on her portfolio, "then I'll start on the last series."

The editor came out from behind her desk to give Carol a peck on the cheek. At the door she asked with perky abruptness, "Who did it, by the way?"

From anyone but the irrepressible Binny, the question would have seemed either crass or merely incomprehensible. But Carol understood.

"They don't know. The police think she was probably killed by a man who's committed a lot of other murders."

Binny gave a low moan. "What a world," she said, "but don't dwell on it too much, pet. Go on, do your work. Take my word, you live under a lucky star and you'll always be fine."

That was a guarantee no one could give. But perhaps because Binny looked so much like a sorceress, Carol liked hearing it and accepted it as the truth.

Waiting for the elevator, she glanced at the glass case in the reception area displaying the most important books published recently by E. B. Fox & Co. It pleased her to see that two of hers—not new, but lately reissued—were included in the selection. Yes, she mused all the way down in the elevator, she had a lucky life.

She had taken only two steps into the lobby when the thought was chased from her mind. In front of a newsstand halfway between her and the street door stood a tall man wearing a dark overcoat and a homburg. His back was to her as he bought a paper, but he was positioned so that he could easily keep an eye on people heading out of the building. She knew at once that it was Paul Miller.

If he had been tracking her today, then the same could be true of yesterday . . . or any day. Yet why, if he was so clever about concealing himself, had she managed to spot him so easily now?

Whatever the answer, Carol didn't want to confront him. She whirled, intending to return upstairs, just as the elevator doors slid shut. None of the other elevators were open.

Tossing a look over her shoulder, Carol saw Miller skimming the newspaper. If he remained distracted for a few seconds more, she might slip past him, screened by people coming in and out. She moved to one side and began walking in measured steps—not running, which would be more likely to attract his attention. Separated by twenty or thirty feet, she came abreast of him, then went past and didn't glance behind her until she had reached the glass revolving door. Only after she was inside, and the door was turning, did she dare a backward glance.

Though still halfway back in the lobby, Miller was already moving rapidly toward the street. Carol leaned harder into the revolving door, burst outside, and started running, dodging through the heavy stream of pedestrians on Madison Avenue. With her large port-folio slapping against her legs, she felt hopelessly clumsy. Her best hope, she decided, was to conceal herself, get out of sight.

Reaching the corner of Fifty-second Street, she checked quickly over her shoulder. He was still fifteen yards away, held back by the thick pedestrian traffic. Darting around the corner, she headed toward Fifth Avenue. At once she saw that the display windows on her right were filled with mannequins wearing colorful women's sportswear. Scurrying through the crowd to the boutique's corner entrance, she dashed inside.

Heedless of the curious stares of shoppers and salesgirls, she raced to the nearest freestanding rack of dresses and ducked down behind it. She parted the hangers a crack and peered through just in time to see Miller racing past the shop window.

Safe for a moment, she thought, even if it might not be long before he doubled back.

"Are you in trouble, miss?"

Carol looked up. A young salesgirl was hovering over her. "Yes, yes, I am," Carol replied breathlessly, still crouching by the rack though she knew she must look foolish. "Can you let me use a phone?"

"There's one over there behind the register."

To use it, Carol saw, she'd have to stand in view of the windows. But if Miller did return and see her, what could he do in the presence of several witnesses?

Leaving her portfolio propped against the rack, Carol went to the cashier's counter, took out her pocket wallet, and found the card Eric Gaines had told her to carry. One of the salesgirls handed her the phone and she dialed.

"One-one-two, Detectives," a voice answered.

"Eric?"

"No. This is Connally. You want Lieutenant Gaines?"

"Yes." *Let him be there,* she prayed silently, and exhaled with relief as she heard the other receiver clunk onto a desk and the voice of the first man echo loudly, "Lieutenant, some broad's on the horn. Sexy voice. Sounds like she's really panting for you, too."

Panting indeed, Carol thought irritably. She snatched a glance toward the big front show windows. Still no sign of Miller.

She turned back to the counter and hunched over, keeping her head down as Eric's voice came on the phone.

"Gaines."

"Thank God. Eric, this is Carol." Her voice broke. "I need help—"

"Okay, Carol, take it easy and just spell it out for me. What's happened?"

"Miller—that crazy man—he's been following me. I had to run into a store to get away from him. That's where I'm—"

"Where is it?" he cut in.

"On the corner of Fifty-second and Madison. A boutique called—" She cast a wild glance across the counter, searching for a receipt with the store's name, but before she found it, one of the salesgirls whispered an answer. She repeated it to Eric. "Pincushion."

"All right, Pincushion, Fifty-second and Mad," he said. "Now, listen: my precinct's in Queens so I can't get there fast enough, but I'll relay this to Midtown South and they'll have a car there in a flash. Just hold tight, kid, and if that nutcase shows up again, stall him and keep him there. Can you handle it?"

"I'll try."

"Good girl."

Carol heard the click of Eric disconnecting. Handing the receiver to the girl at the counter, she suddenly became aware that all the women in the store were staring at her.

"I'm fine," she announced distractedly to the salespeople and the customers. "That was the police; they told me to wait here. But you just . . . do whatever you have to do."

At the mention of the police the loose circle of women quickly pulled away, moving in a pack to the door and out to the street.

"Jesus," one of the salesgirls said. "What the hell . . . ?"

"I'm sorry," Carol said nervously, "I didn't mean to cause trouble, but this man . . ."

She hadn't moved from the counter before Miller appeared outside, stepping into the frame of one of the large windows like a villain arriving onstage from the wings. Frozen in her tracks, she watched as he scanned up and down the street . . . until he turned around and saw her.

"Oh God." The small cry emerged unbidden from her lips, a reflex call for help.

Miller had pushed through the door and was coming toward her, his hands raised as if in benediction, a calming gesture obviously meant to preempt any panic.

"Carol, please listen," he appealed, "I need to talk to you again—"

"Stay away," she shouted, almost adding that the police were coming any second. Then she remembered Eric's instruction: stall.

"There's no need to be afraid, Carol," he said. "I'm not going to hurt you." He continued moving forward with slower, smaller steps, but no less deliberately.

"Mr. Miller, we've talked enough. Just leave me alone."

"I can't, Carol. There's something only you can help me with—a problem with my investigation."

He was within ten feet now, advancing with the same

careful pace in which a rescuer might approach someone poised to jump off a bridge.

"What problem?" she asked. She edged off to one side, moving to put one of the racks between them.

"We'll talk about it. But not here. Trust me, that's all I ask, give me a few more minutes of your time." He threw a glance of appeal at the salespeople, who were edging away, not wanting to get involved. "Please don't be alarmed, ladies," he assured them in his courtly way, dressing it up with a smile. "We'll have this all straightened out in a minute." He moved closer, extending his hand. "Now, Carol, let's go have a cup of coffee somewhere."

How in hell did she keep stalling him? Try on a dress? Ask him if he liked it? An unthinking reflex sent her bolting for the door. She reached the exit several paces ahead of him and was still in front when she made it into the street. But opening the door had cost her time, and Miller was at her heels. She moved only another two paces before she felt her arm snagged in his grip. Spinning around, she raised her free hand in the air, balled into a fist.

But before she could swing it down against his face, she heard the sirens, and it seemed like only a moment later that the blue-and-white car veered over to the sidewalk, bumping straight up over the curb so that the fender came to a halt only inches from Miller.

Two policemen exploded out of its front doors. Miller let go, but even as he was grabbed roughly by one of the policemen, he didn't turn from Carol.

"This is the man!" she called out loudly, pointing at Miller. "He was following me, chasing me."

The other policeman ran to Carol's side. "You the lady who called Detective Gaines, one hundred and twelfth precinct?"

"Yes," she gasped with relief.

"All right, miss, you wait here. Another car'll be here in a minute to take you downtown." The police-

man nodded to the officer who was holding Miller.
"Read him his rights and get his ass outta here."

Miller continued gazing at Carol as the officer rapidly intoned the Miranda rights to remain silent and
have counsel.

"I'm sorry you felt this was necessary," Miller said
softly to Carol when the policeman had finished. "But
I understand." He smiled at her, and then, with an impressive show of strength, jerked his arm free of the
cop's grasp . . . so that he could lift his hand to give
Carol a courtly tip of his homburg.

8 "YOU LET HIM GO?" Carol pulled forward on her chair and gave Eric a despairing look.

"It wasn't up to me, Carol," Eric replied. "It's not my precinct." He was poised on the edge of a scarred wooden conference table—except for the four chairs placed around it, the only furniture in the bare dingy room on the ground floor of the police station.

"Let him go," Carol repeated, shaking her head in disbelief. "How could they?" She had spent an hour sitting in the precinct's waiting area, and all that time she had imagined that Miller was being interrogated and booked.

Eric leaned over from his higher perch. "Carol, there weren't grounds for an arrest. Running after a woman to talk to her isn't a crime. He didn't assault you—"

"He grabbed me when I was leaving the store."

"That's tough to prosecute," Eric said forcefully. "Maybe we could get him on assault if you swore out a complaint. But as it is, we were pushing it a little to bring Miller in. Strictly speaking, the officers should've *asked* him to accompany them; it should have been 'a voluntary.' "

Frustrated beyond words, Carol looked away toward the room's only window, a large grimy pane protected by steel bars. This was ludicrous. Here she was feeling like a prisoner—hostage to a stranger's craziness—while Miller had been set free.

She turned back to Eric. "I don't understand this,"

she said, working to keep a level tone. "You know that there's some man walking around loose, a man who's killed again and again and again—killed women like me—a man who's able to pass himself off as reasonable. And then this man Miller starts bothering me, telling lies to explain his interest in me and in all these murders . . . and all you can say is he has to be treated with kid gloves because he did nothing wrong, as if he were perfectly *harmless*." She gave a half-laugh, then her voice cracked as the edge of real hysteria broke through. "What the hell is going on?" she added, crying it to the ceiling.

Eric slid off the desk and crouched beside her, a coach in pep-talk position. "Carol, honey, believe me, if I thought it was going to put you in serious danger . . ."

She lifted her eyes to his. "How can you be sure Miller isn't dangerous?"

"His credentials were checked. He *is* licensed as a private investigator."

Carol gave a twitch of impatience. "For heaven's sake, I saw his license—he told me himself it's not hard to get. And even real policemen have been known to commit murder. License or not, Eric, Miller *did* lie to me: he wasn't hired by the Bonfarros to work on their daughter's case."

Eric's dark eyebrows were bridged with concern. "Carol, what can I do? It may be wrong to tell lies—but it's no crime. Miller knows the law, too. All he'd show us was his investigator's license. The address filed with the state is a security firm in Connecticut, and they wouldn't tell us anything."

"You mean you don't even know where he lives?"

Eric stood up. "He told us no more than he was required to tell—and then he threatened to sue for false arrest if we booked him. Which we couldn't." Eric walked away to the window and stared out. "I went too far—sending a couple of squad cars. There just wasn't sufficient cause. And Miller knew it."

There was a silence. "Are you in trouble for helping me?" Carol asked.

He turned back to her. "No, I can take care of precinct politics. But there's something else: the order to let Miller go came from upstairs, command level. He made one phone call after he walked in here . . . and half an hour later the word came down."

"What does that mean?" Carol asked.

Eric shrugged, took a step toward her. "Could be anything. Maybe he's got a powerful lawyer. Or friends in high places . . . or maybe even somebody wants him loose—with a tail on him—so he can be kept under surveillance."

Carol stiffened. "In other words, he might be a killer."

"It's not impossible. But if that was the case, you'd be safer than any ordinary Jane Doe out there in the street. Because the somebody who gave the orders would probably be the Feds—FBI—and whether or not you could spot it, Carol, there'd be surveillance on this guy tighter than a flea's ass." Hastily he tacked on, " 'Scuse me—cop talk."

She stood up. "Well, however I feel about it, I guess I don't have any choice but to live with it. Or," she added tartly, "die with it."

Eric crossed the last gap of floor between them. "Carol, I'll say it again: I'm not going to let anything bad happen to you."

In his stance and the husky timbre of his voice, she sensed more than a promise of safety. His desire for her was suddenly almost palpable in the air around them.

"How about if I drive you home?" he asked.

"Yes, I'd appreciate that."

*   *   *

Riding in the unmarked black police sedan, they kept to small talk. Eric's father, Carol learned, had been an elementary school principal, retired now, and his mother was a piano teacher. Both parents had urged their son, who was eager to join the Army, to attend college instead. Eric had gone from high school to the University of Wisconsin on an athletic scholarship in track and field.

". . . pole vault and fifty-yard dash," he was saying, just as they pulled up at a hydrant beside the entrance to Carol's apartment house.

He turned off the engine. Neither of them moved.

"Official car," he said. "I can park by a hydrant for as long as I want."

She smiled at him and put her hand on his sleeve. "I like you, Eric. But let's not move too fast." Leaning across the seat, she kissed him on the lips and yielded quickly when he pulled her closer.

"That was nice," he said. "I'd like to see you again soon, Carol."

She nodded. "Give me a few days, though. I have a lot of work, a deadline."

"I'll call on the weekend."

She got out, turned back for a little wave, and then went into her building. From the elevator, before the doors closed, she could see that Eric was still parked outside.

On an impulse, after walking into her apartment, she went out onto the terrace and leaned over the railing to look down at the street. Eric's car was still there.

And again, when she looked five minutes later.

She changed into her terry robe and glanced idly over some of her day's work at the drawing table. Then she went back outside for another look. The space at the hydrant stood empty.

Had he stayed those few minutes for surveillance? Perhaps he was more worried than he'd been willing to admit.

*   *   *

In the middle of the next morning her bottle of india ink ran dry. It was a miserable day out, rain hammering down in sheets against the windows. Carol searched the house in vain for more of the thick black drawing ink—anything to stay inside. But at last she surrendered. She excavated her galoshes from the back of the coat closet, slipped on her yellow oilskin sou'wester, and set out for the art store, several blocks away.

Once she was slogging through the rain, she was happy with her choice. The downpour was the worst the city had seen in weeks, so that there was a sense of adventure in being among the few hardy souls on the street. At Jensen's, the art store, she bought not one bottle of ink but two, telling herself that the next time her supplies ran out it might be in the middle of a blizzard.

Just as she finished paying for her purchase, the shower got even heavier, coming down in huge gobs as though a bucket in the sky had been overturned. Carol hunched down to shield her face from the pelting rain before charging out into the street, and she had gone only a few feet when she butted up against someone coming in the other direction. "Oh, sorry," she said, lifting her head.

When she saw that it was Paul Miller in front of her, she was too stunned to move.

He held her in a riveting gaze, hands stuffed into the pockets of his overcoat. Channeled by the rim of his tilted homburg, rain dripped in a stream from one side of the hat onto his shoulder. When he spoke, it was with a burning conviction she had never heard in the voice of any other man.

"Miss Warren, I swear to you by everything that's holy: I mean you no harm."

If it had been a sunny day, perhaps she would have run. But the rain falling around them was like a curtain of fine silver pins, walling them into a small private compound.

"What do you want, Mr. Miller?" she said quietly. "For God's sake, tell me what you want."

A look of tremendous sadness swept across his stolid features. "It can't be put off any longer," he said. "But suppose we go somewhere out of the rain. That coffee shop . . ."

He gestured with only a nod to the far side of the street, keeping his hands in his pockets as though being careful to avoid any movement that might threaten her.

She thought of Eric saying that either Miller was safe or was being kept under tight surveillance. Glancing toward the coffee shop, Carol shifted her eyes in all directions, hoping to see some subtle sign of protection. Of course there was nothing but a city street under a downpour. The man huddled in a doorway on the opposite sidewalk could be a plainclothes observer—or just someone waiting for a bus.

Miller was waiting for her answer, a statue in the rain.

All the while she was crossing the street, entering the luncheonette, letting him help her out of her sou'wester, Carol told herself she was a fool. Still, an ember of intuition kept glowing beneath the dark thoughts. It was far from impossible that Miller's air of genteel basic decency was a well-rehearsed pose. Yet something told her he deserved one more chance, that there had been some solid reason for his lie—and at the least she wanted to have that riddle answered.

They settled in a booth, facing each other. Carol said nothing as Miller gave the waitress the most perfunctory order. "Just two coffees."

When the waitress left, he glanced to the paper bag Carol had set down at one side of the table. "Takes a real professional to venture out on a day like this for such a small purchase. What did you buy?"

"Ink," she said shortly. "Look, Mr. Miller, we're way past the point where we can . . . normalize relations. There's nothing normal about the way you've followed me, and the pretenses you've—"

"Pretenses?" he interrupted. "I know there are things I've held back, but whatever I've told you has been true."

"Even your story about the Bonfarros?" she cut in. "I called that poor girl's mother, and she said she'd never hired any private investigator."

"And I never claimed she did. I'm terribly sorry if you got the wrong impression. What I recall telling you is that I knew she and her husband were very dissatisfied with the police investigation . . . and also that it was about the same time their daughter disappeared that I came into the case."

His eyes looked steadily into hers, almost daring her to refute him. She thought back to their lunch; in the whole inventory of phrases raked up from memory, she realized there was none that actually stated he had been hired by the victim's family. She'd made that connection herself.

Yet there beyond the challenge in his steady gaze, she saw again the shrewd intelligence. It made her suspect he might have contrived to create the very misunderstanding he now lamented.

And there was something else. "You told me a letter was found in Anne's purse. I know that's a lie."

"I'm sorry about that," Miller replied. "I was mistaken. There was a letter, but it wasn't found in her purse. It was in her desk at work."

Could that be true? Even if it was, she felt that every move Miller made had been contrived to keep her off balance.

Why all this clever maneuvering?

The waitress brought two coffees. Both went untouched.

Abruptly Miller resumed, speaking now with the cool declaratory tone of a lecturer. "In the past two years, Miss Warren, I have traveled more than eighty thousand miles, crisscrossing New York again and again and the states bordering it—New Jersey, Connecticut, Pennsylvania. I have also taken several trips to more distant parts of the country. I have done nothing but work on this single series of murders—trying to pick up a clue, any small shred of evidence that might lead to identifying the man the police call the Deep Woods Killer." Sensitive to Carol's glance of inquiry, he explained, "The name comes from the fact that, so far, all the bodies that have been recovered were found in wooded areas, always way off the beaten track." He paused, apparently to allow for questions, but she held back, more curious as to how he would continue. "The man we're chasing is unquestionably one of the most vicious and intelligent ever sought in the history of law enforcement, here or anywhere else. Police departments in several states and a dozen municipalities are at work on this case, spending millions in money and manpower, and all these bloodhounds are still chasing their own tails more than sniffing at the guilty man's heels." He laid his arms flat on the table and leaned across to her. "And then there's me," he went on, "out there on my own, following my own hunches, scraping around in the muddy footprints the clumsy crowd leaves behind, looking for what they've forgotten . . . or were too monkey-brained stupid to see."

For the first time Carol heard Miller's tone of quiet control give way to a quaver of anger. But when he resumed only a moment later, the faint thunder had rolled away. "And so they have their ideas, and I have mine. Sometimes we converge, sometimes we don't. But I keep going my own way, because I don't care if they do it or I do it . . . but this monster has got to be caught." He paused once more to engage her eyes, then added, "Doesn't he?"

He waited now, as if he really needed to hear the answer, no matter how curiously unnecessary the question.

"Of course," Carol replied. "There's no argument about that. It's the way you've—"

He spoke right over her. "I haven't wanted to tell you more until now, Miss Warren, because I kept hoping it wouldn't be necessary. But there really isn't any way around it now. I need all the help I can get, every edge. I can't refuse to take even the smallest advantage."

There was a sense of yearning in his voice that actually moved Carol. "As long as it's the truth, Mr. Miller, just tell me what it is, and I'll try to help."

The smile that touched his lips came from the gratitude of a needy man, the smile a beggar might give when a coin was dropped into his cap. "It's taken a long time," he said, "endless traveling, talking to endless numbers of people, but I've got a list now of seventy-three men who qualify as suspects for various reasons. Because they fit some of the descriptions we've got—sketchy as they are—or because their jobs took them over the whole area where these crimes occurred, or they owned the kind of car that a witness saw parked somewhere near the place a body was found. The clues are minimal usually, everything has to be cross-checked against everything else. But these seventy-three men are the only ones whose names have come up, and who haven't yet been ruled out. I'm convinced one of them is the Deep Woods Killer."

Carol stared at him. Even without any experience of detective work, she knew that Miller was deluding himself if he thought he was anywhere near solving the case. Seventy-three suspects? By Miller's own admission, even those who were listed had been targeted by the most insubstantial information—vague clues, sketchy descriptions. How real, indeed, was the list he spoke about?

She couldn't help wondering again if Miller was, in some way, a disturbed person. Not the killer; she believed that working on the case could simply be his job. But however the job had come to him, she guessed that it had evolved into something more—an obsession.

He had let the silence continue.

"And what do you want from me?" Carol asked.

"I want to know everything you can tell me about one of the men on the list."

"Why me?"

"Because," Miller replied, "he's someone you know."

Carol regarded him skeptically.

"It's a long shot," Miller went on. "But even the littlest thing you tell me might throw some light in a corner and show up something crucial."

"About whom," she asked. "Who is it, Mr. Miller?"

His hesitation seemed endless. "This is very hard for me. But, you understand, it has to be done."

"I understand," Carol replied impatiently. "Just tell me, damn it. Tell me what you need, so I can . . . get on with my life." She grabbed up the package of ink on the table as though preparing to leave.

Miller nodded quickly, ducking his eyes so that again he had that aspect of an obedient schoolboy. "The man I need to ask you about," he said finally, "is your brother."

She could not say how long his last words went on echoing in her brain—two seconds or two minutes—but for the whole time her emotions went reeling through a chaotic series of changes. Shock to anger to pity to dread to grief to simple amazement. And at the end of the avalanche of feelings there was nothing but a settling calm. She considered calmly whether to ask if she had heard him correctly . . . and then calmly answered it herself. Of course she had; if he actually had Tommy on his list of suspects, then that could most easily explain the reason he had been stalking her. Would even explain his reluctance to tell her the truth.

But being able to rationalize this much of what Miller had done did not in anyway soften her reaction to what he had charged.

"Mr. Miller," she said with great reserve, "you still haven't told me who you're working for, and why, if you suspect my brother, you're following me, not him. It can't be that you want to keep him from knowing your suspicions—because you ought to realize I'll certainly call him and—"

"I told you who I was working for," Miller interrupted. "I work on my own. And I have checked on your brother's movements. As for calling him, of course I understand you'd want to do that."

"You work on your own," Carol shot back. "But for *whom?*"

"For me."

She stared at him, trying to work out what he meant. Could he give all this time to it purely as some kind of personal quest?

"So you, on your own," she said—still calm, but with traces of acid beginning to show in her tone— "and working from the thinnest evidence, you've decided that my brother could be guilty of . . . of crimes like these."

"He's on a list of suspects, Miss Warren. That's all I said. But whoever is on that list, I don't intend to leave them alone, to leave any question about them unanswered." He gazed at her steadily, the vow restated in his eyes.

Then her mind flipped, and fury overtook her. Her hand went to the cup of black coffee, and she had an urge to throw the still steaming black liquid in his face.

But this demon, too, she throttled down. To show any loss of control, it occurred to her, might even reflect on Tommy, be taken as evidence of some violent strain in the family.

Gathering up her package of ink, she slid out of the booth and stood in one quick, smooth motion.

Miller brought his head up sharply, obviously taken by surprise.

"I have only one piece of information to give you, Mr. Miller. You're way out of line to have my brother on your list. It's a mistake that has now caused me a great deal of pain—not because I doubt my brother, but because of the way you've acted. But I'm going to assume it's over now. I can't keep you from having your list, or bothering other people with it. All I care about is that you don't bother me again. Have I made myself clear, Mr. Miller? Leave me alone, or by God I'll make certain that you suffer for what you're doing."

She was already turning to walk away as he replied quietly, "I suffer now, dear girl."

These words, too, never stopped echoing in her mind as she walked home through the merciless rain.

9 TOMMY? A KILLER?

No, not merely that—but the most 'depraved butcher.

Carol spun away from the phone and returned to her drawing board, where the face of tiny Dana stared back at her with its unformed eyes and unpainted hair. Sketching the outlines of the vulture poised to strike the child—indeed, creating any imaginary beasts— seemed ridiculous. Carol couldn't seem to make them less threatening, as Binny had asked, and she had her own monster to cope with, a lunatic named Paul Miller insinuating himself into her life. Telling monstrous lies.

She'd tried to reach Tommy, but he had not been at his office, and she was afraid to call him at home. Suppose Jill answered. Carol worried that her voice would give her away, that Jill might detect trouble. But she had to talk with someone about Miller.

Unthinkingly she slapped her brush down—and then cursed herself: a slash of red had destroyed Dana's face; the mouth now opening into a scream that appeared to spew blood. And at that moment the features shifted before Carol's eyes and became Anne Donaldson.

Was that it? Was that what had linked Tommy to Miller's investigation, the fact that he had known Anne? But Tommy wouldn't have known all those other women. The thoughts went round and round, speculations that made no sense. Christ, wasn't it absurd even to be weighing the pros and cons of suspicion?

Carol stood, went into the kitchen, and poured a glass of club soda. She glanced into the hallway at three framed prints hanging on the wall. At the publication party for her first book, her friend Margot Jenner had given her the delicately tinted etchings—St. Nicholas, St. Francis de Sales, and St. Luke, the patron saints of children, writers, and artists. Although not a Catholic, Carol found herself hoping that the saints were watching over her now.

She went to the refrigerator. Stuck to the door with a magnet was Eric Gaines's card. She picked up the wall phone.

Eric, thankfully, was at his precinct. Hearing his voice, Carol could feel some of the tension leave her body.

"Hi, Carol. Anything wrong?"

She forced an offhand tone. "No, but I have a favor to ask?"

"Name it."

"It's a big one, and it may seem a little strange. But I wouldn't ask unless—"

"I want to help any way I can," Eric cut in. "Shoot."

Okay, here goes, she actually said in her mind, priming herself. "Is there a list of suspects in the Donaldson case—I mean, all those cases you think are connected?"

Eric's answer came slowly. "Yes . . ."

She paused again. Her throat had gone dry. "I know this is unusual, but would it be possible for me to see it?"

"Oh, Carol," he started to object, "I never thought—"

"Look, I'm not asking you to give me a copy," she hurried on. "It would be enough if you'd just read it to me, give me the names." She heard a faintly whining ring in her voice and she hated it, but if it would get through to him . . .

"Hold on a second," he said. Waiting, Carol stretched the phone cord to the window, feeling the need for air, and in a moment Eric returned. "I could get in major trouble," he said evenly, "breaking the regs like this. Anyway, the computer's down, so I don't have them in alphabetical order. I'll read you the labels on the files. Do you want first names, too?"

"No, last names will be fine."

"When I'm done, I hope you'll tell me what this is all about." Eric started reading. "McCrory, Brown, Lewis, Donovan, Avery . . ."

Carol listened intently, gripping the phone—her lifeline to peace of mind. The names went by, one after the other, names of unknown men—other innocents, of course, almost every one had to be. And it hit her then, as it hadn't in the past hour—the madness of Miller's charge, the utter magnitude of it.

". . . Boardman, Esteban, Smith, Pelletier, Ramirez, Davis, Ogden, another Smith, Canetti . . ."

She wanted to interrupt Eric, urge him to go faster, but she feared breaking the spell. He might well decide to stop altogether.

". . . Woznicki, Peck, Cohen, Springmeyer . . ." Eric stopped reading. "That's it, Carol, that's all of them."

"Thank God," she said with a sigh.

"Now tell me," Eric said. "What's going on, Carol? What were you expecting?"

"I just thought that maybe . . . maybe somebody I knew might be on it."

"Who?" Eric asked. "Carol, for chrissakes, if you know anything about this case and you're not telling me . . ."

She didn't want to reveal more but felt she had no choice. Eric had helped her. Could she refuse an explanation? "I wanted to be sure that . . . one of the names wasn't . . . my brother's."

"Why on earth would you think that?"

Carol admitted then that she had talked with Miller again. "He has a new story now," she explained. "He told me that he has a list of suspects in the case—and one of them is my brother."

"Jesus!" Eric exclaimed. "Carol, whatever this guy's up to, our investigation is the official one, and your brother's not a suspect."

"You can't imagine what this is like, it's so awful—"

"Hey, hon', I do understand. Are you going to be okay? I get off at seven, I could stop by . . ."

"No, thank you, I just needed some reassurance. You've given me that, and I'm grateful."

Eric made her promise that if she was still upset she would let him know. His concern soothed her, and after she hung up the black cloud that Miller had left hovering over her lifted.

Instead of working she sat at her desk and answered adoring fan letters from children. What joy they gave her, and what pleasure she gained from answering them. But today her heart wasn't in it, and she had written only five notes before she started glancing at the phone, wanting to try to reach Tommy again.

Yet no matter how many times she doodled the Saddle River number on the paper in front of her, she couldn't bring herself to make the call.

"Carol, wait there, will you? I'll be down in a minute."

The voice through the intercom sounded agitated. Carol went back out to the sidewalk in front of the Greenwich Village apartment building where her friend Margot Jenner lived. In two minutes Margot and her husband Larry came through the lobby door. Despite the faint dark circles under Larry's eyes, he carried himself with verve. The sturdy Englishman, Margot called him. He had a large square-jawed face and wiry salt-and-pepper hair.

"Carol, how good to see you," he said cheerfully,

giving her a peck on the cheek. "Why haven't we heard from you? Don't be a reclusive artist. You know what Dr. Johnson said: Friendship is in need of constant repair."

Larry Jenner really was a rock of strength, Carol thought. Out of work for six months and still chipper as ever. She forced a smile. "I guess I've been a little preoccupied."

"You must come up to the country some weekend," he offered. "The leaves are putting on their annual show." He touched Margot's hand and started toward Broadway. "I'll get the papers. You two have a good chat."

Carol and Margot walked across University Place toward Fifth Avenue. Ten years ago they had met in a figure drawing class at the Art Students League. Back then, Margot was a rebellious belle from Memphis come north to be a serious painter. But while Carol had succeeded with her children's books, Margot was mostly ignored by the art world's power brokers. Then came her first big show—and a *Times* review that dismissed her work with one insult after another: empty, derivative, jejune.

Margot sank into a year-long depression—until, thank God, she met Larry Jenner. With him she had built a domestic life in which her view of herself as a success or failure didn't depend on art critics.

"Larry seems really well," Carol observed.

"Yeah, he's like the autumn leaves," Margot replied dourly. "He puts on a good show. I woke up this morning and he was crying in the corner of the bedroom. The truth is, he's at his wit's end."

"My God, he could've fooled me." Carol stopped. "If this is an inconvenient time—"

"No, let's get something to eat, I needed to get out of the house."

They continued toward Fifth Avenue. Margot, wearing a bright patterned sweater and trim black slacks,

looked her usual fashionable self, and at the corner
a leering construction worker called out, "Hey, babe,
nice tits!"

Carol had learned to brush off the city's crude street
talk. But Margot wheeled on the man. "If you had any
style," she said sweetly, "do you know what you'd do?
You'd go fuck yourself."

As they walked on, Margot sighed. "All these years
of feminism and we still have to put up with jerks treating us like Playboy bunnies." She took a breath. "I'm
irritable, that's all. Larry thought he had a new job but
this morning it fell through."

Larry Jenner had been a successful stock analyst
until his firm laid off three thousand employees last
spring. To make matters worse, Margot now told
Carol, Larry's first wife, mother of his two children,
had been admitted to Bellevue last week suffering a
nervous breakdown.

"God only knows what all of this is doing to the
kids," Margot went on. "They're obviously upset, and
one way they show it is by treating me like a dog. Let
me tell you, being a stepmother is *exactly* what it's
cracked up to be." She rounded the corner, heading
downtown. "Larry's climbing the walls, too. We're
eating up big chunks of our savings."

"It's natural to be upset," Carol offered.

"Upset? Larry's unfathomably depressed, Carol.
It's one of the burdens of being a man—if you can't
support your family, you feel useless—but I worry
sometimes about what he might do."

What did she mean? That he might commit suicide?
Or just walk away from the pressures . . . ?

At Eighth Street they went into One Fifth, a restaurant with ship's paneling on the walls and amber-lit
sconces in the form of portholes. The maître d' led
them to a table facing the street. "I'm behaving terribly," Margot said, sitting down. "You wanted to talk
to me and all I've done is gab about my problems."

Carol had no desire to add to Margot's troubles by revealing her own. Mechanically she started talking about Tommy's housewarming, the fun she'd had, her date with Frank Matheson.

"He actually bought you dinner?" Margot said brightly. "That's a good sign. Most of them want to be modern and split the check." She flagged a waiter and both she and Carol ordered croissants and coffee. Then Margot sat back and folded her hands. "Now let's have it. You said you needed my li'l ol' shoulder to lean on."

Carol kneaded the edge of the linen tablecloth between her thumb and forefinger, then told Margot about Paul Miller, his investigation of a serial killer, and all his lies.

"Bizarre," Margot said. "What the hell does the guy want?"

"You're not going to believe this, but he says Tommy's a suspect."

"Carol . . . you're joking."

"I wish I were," Carol said, her voice sinking. She started to say more, then stopped.

"Darlin', something else is chewing at you. What is it?"

What indeed? It was only now, confronted with the question, that Carol was able to articulate an answer. "It's terrible to say this, but a couple times today I thought maybe I don't really know Tommy." As Carol heard her own words, a wave of emotional exhaustion rolled over her. She rested her forehead on her palm, stunned at the enormity of what she had just admitted.

Margot grasped Carol's shoulder. "Take it easy. You're blowing this way out of the park. This fellow Miller, what did he say? He's got seventy-odd suspects, right?"

Carol nodded.

"Okay, so seventy people seem to have some link to this. But except for one of them, they're all innocent. For that matter, maybe *every* one is innocent. Miller's not a cop, you don't know what he is. When you get down to it, his list doesn't mean diddly. You've already heard from this cop in Queens that Tommy isn't on his list—the *real* list."

God bless Margot. She made perfect sense, and Carol was suddenly ashamed of herself—ashamed at this defection of the heart from her own brother. "You're right," she said.

"You bet I am. Still, you've ought to pin this Miller fella down. Who is he? What does he really want? Something here ain't square, darlin'. He gets your handwriting, but his explanation is baloney. He tells you some family is paying him, but it turns out they aren't. For your sake, and for Tommy's, find out who he is."

Margot was like an antidote to a powerful poison, and for the first time in days Carol felt she could see clearly. Fragile in the wake of Anne's death, she had simply allowed herself to be swept up in a stranger's delusions.

As soon as she got home, she went to the kitchen and dialed the Meditron offices again. No answer. Of course, it was already past six.

She decided to risk trying Tommy at home.

It was Jill who answered, cheerfully pleased to hear from her. Hadn't the housewarming been great? Yes, Carol agreed, wonderful, the house looked splendid.

"And what about Frank Matheson?" Jill asked. "Have you seen him? Tom's very fond of him, you know."

She'd had a delightful evening with Frank, Carol confided, and to herself thought how well she was performing. If there was anything strained in her voice, Jill hadn't picked up on it. "Is Tommy home?" she asked then. "There are a couple of things I wanted to speak to him about."

"Oh, didn't he mention that he was going to Washington? He's seeing some money people down there. If it's important, I can give you the number of his hotel."

"No," Carol said, "it can wait." She was wary of unsettling Jill, and more important, of disturbing Tommy in the midst of business negotiations. Yet she couldn't resist a doubting question. "How's Tommy been feeling? I mean, about the company? He's not looking for investors in Washington because there's any trouble . . . ?"

"No, things are going well," Jill said. "I think we did a good job of impressing his backers at the party. *You* were certainly a big hit, Carol. It makes Tom look good to have a famous sister. After you left he was thinking maybe you could sign some books as Christmas gifts for his clients."

"I'd be glad to," Carol said. "It's nice to hear Tommy's in good spirits."

There was a pause as if Jill were actually weighing her comment. "Sometimes he does seem a little overworked," she said, "distracted, you know, worried about sales and things like that. But otherwise he hasn't been this happy in years."

Carol said she was pleased to hear it and remarked that the effects of success on Jill, too, seemed terrific.

"That's true," Jill said. "It wasn't easy when we were short of money. But now . . . well, I never thought I'd enjoy school this much. Everything is so good, Carol, I keep expecting something terrible to happen. That's neurotic, isn't it? Always expecting to be punished for being happy."

"I know the feeling," Carol said, then told Jill she would try Tommy next week.

After hanging up she went into the living room and sank into the overstuffed club chair. Six days ago, she thought, a woman disappeared in Brooklyn. Vanished into the night from a parking lot. And Tommy is fine. Happier than ever.

But damn it, why shouldn't he be? Carol heard Margot's voice in her head: *Seventy suspects? Except for one, they're all innocent . . . maybe every one is innocent.* Yes, all of them, Carol thought. Every last one.

IN THE DEEP WOODS

This one, he thought, was very brave.

Some surrendered early, some struggled even after he had gotten them tied up, gag in place, but they used up their strength quickly and then became quiet and resigned. With this one there had been tears at first, but they had flowed from eyes that were wide and glaring—tears of rage and frustration rather than of fear and grief for the anticipated loss of her own life. And the walk into the woods hadn't been easy at all, far from it. Even trussed up completely, she had never for a minute given up struggling, knees and elbows pummeling his chest and sides as he carried her over his shoulder.

Now she was on the ground; but not, as many did, simply waiting it out anxiously, moaning or crying or praying, or lying back in surrender with eyes closed, pretending it was a dream— or trying to avoid seeing his preparations. He had seen a lot of different reactions. But none exactly like this.

She sat up in the pile of leaves he had gathered—his improvised altar—her legs pulled up under her as she stared at him with angry eyes, their burning ferocity accented by the redness left from the tears that had now stopped. Even though he had already scissored away the blouse and bra, had laid the oilskin packet on the ground where she could see it, still she hadn't rearranged herself instinctively into some shrinking posture, wasn't cringing. He smiled as it occurred to him that maybe it wasn't merely that she was brave. . . .

Maybe she wasn't normal.

He took the pack of cigarettes from his shirt pocket, tapped one out, and lit it with a match. He didn't blow out the flame immediately but held the match in his hand like a tiny torch.

For the past few minutes he had been leaning against a tree, just trading stares, but now he took a few steps toward her.

Her eyes widened slightly, but he still didn't see any expression of outright dread.

"Burning to death," he said, "is a horrible way to die." He switched his gaze between the flame and the pile of leaves on which she was perched. She stiffened, lifted her chin, but what he saw was still something less than terror. Her eyebrows creased, as if she was trying to comprehend what he had said, why he would say it.

He smiled. "You know me too well," he said, "don't you?" He blew out the match then, crumbled the end, and put the wooden shaft into his pocket. "You know I wouldn't do that."

Careful not to inhale the smoke, he took a long puff on the cigarette, watching from the corner of his eye as the ash glowed red. He moved up next to her, then took the cigarette from his mouth, and in a quick deft movement touched the burning end to the tip of one of her nipples. A muffled squeal came through the gag, and her body jolted backward, but he was prepared for her retreat, so that he was able to keep the singeing ash pressed against her breast. The amber tissue was burned to black.

He pulled the cigarette away, but her whimpering squeal went on. That was better, he thought. She even sounded like a pig about to be slaughtered.

He went back to where the oilskin packet lay, walked around it so that she would have a view of what he was doing, and knelt down. Untying the string, he opened the flaps. Then he picked up each item—needlessly really, just straightening them or moving them a little farther apart, like a host fussing with the settings at a dinner party. The knives, the saw, the drill, the screwdriver, the long rubber cylinder, and of course the gloves. Until he had finished fiddling, he didn't look at her again.

At last the tone of her cry changed from a squeal of pain to the muffled plea for pity. She was looking at him. And, he was relieved to see, the terror was there. She was normal, after all.

He put on the gloves and passed his hand uncertainly over the different tools, hesitating over his choice. At last he picked up the rubber cylinder and took the scissors again from his pocket.

"Well," he said, as if they were simply going on a picnic, "I think it's about time we got started. . . ."

Her throat flexed with the effort of a scream that puffed out the front of the gag. And though she couldn't possibly articulate a word, he thought he knew exactly what she must be saying.

"Yes," he mocked her as he rolled her over on her stomach. "Pretty please with sugar on it."

10 LIGHT SPARKLED FROM THE SILVER blade of the razor as it sliced across flesh.

"His hands were quick, his fingers strong . . . ," the man's voice sang out. "See your razor gleam."

As Sweeney Todd slashed the snake-oil salesman's throat, a stream of blood squirted onto the stage. Carol had to avert her eyes. Even though it was only theater, it was horrible.

Frank Matheson's invitation had come at the last minute. He had tickets for the City Opera revival of *Sweeney Todd*—bought for out-of-town clients now stuck between planes in Chicago. Having missed the original Broadway hit, Carol immediately accepted. But it wasn't only the show that had lured her. Some time with Frank, she thought, might provide an opportunity to reassure herself about Tommy.

Sitting in the theater, however, the evening felt like a mistake. The Sondheim music was beautiful, but a spectacle about a deranged barber who slit his customer's throats, and his lady friend who chopped them up and baked them into pies, wasn't Carol's idea of entertainment. At times she could keep a distance, but then the gore would overwhelm her and another dark looming figure, more terrifying than the one on stage, would appear in her mind . . . Paul Miller, bringing his accusation against Tommy.

After the show, over drinks at The Ginger Man, Frank was full of praise for the musical. "What's astounding is how it uses murder as a metaphor. Mrs. Lovett bakes pies for Sweeney because she's lonely, she only wants love. Maybe I'm reaching too far, but isn't it about what people to do each other—the cruelties of everyday life—committed in the name of love?"

It was an interpretation, Carol thought, that she wouldn't have been likely to make. Despite Frank's well-practiced performance as a smoothie, he kept showing a thoughtful, intellectual side as well.

"Maybe it's about how Sweeney makes other people suffer for what's been done to him," she said. "Or it's just a scary story to keep us afraid of the dark."

"And afraid of barbers," Frank said with a laugh. "Well, we've come a long way from *Hello, Dolly.*" He looked around at the others in the restaurant. "I love this," he said, "the bustle of an after-theater crowd. And Tom thought I'd hate living in the city."

"He's not one for crowds himself," Carol said, pleased to change the subject. "When we were were teenagers living on Long Island, I liked to come into the city for museums and movies and stuff, but he was happy to stay at home."

"And even then he probably figured you were wrong—though from what I know about Tom, I'll bet he encouraged you to be yourself, do things your own way."

Carol nodded, impressed by Frank's insight into her relationship with Tommy. "Is he like that in the office, too?"

"Yep. If you were cynical, you'd call it management style."

"And," Carol asked wryly, "are you cynical?"

"Not about Tom. He's done a lot for me. I was just a sales manager, and he had faith in me, brought me up the ladder with him."

"You've known him a long time now."

"It's really since he started Meditron that I can call him a friend. At our old jobs we weren't in the office together that much. Though even then I knew he was headed for bigger things."

"How?"

"He just had an air about him," Frank said.

"An air of what?"

Frank gave Carol a curious glance. "Say, how come all these questions about Tom?"

"He's my brother," she replied. "I'm interested."

"But you should know him better than I do."

"Of course I know certain things about him better than anyone." Carol hesitated. "But not . . . his professional life, how he handles the people who work for him, how he . . ." She was lost for a moment, wondering in fact how much there was she didn't know.

Frank studied her. "What's wrong, Carol?"

She tried a smile, but it came across stiffly. "Why do you think something's wrong?"

"Intuition, I guess. Not strictly a feminine trait, you know."

She gazed back at Frank and decided again that she liked what she saw. And so without further anxiety about the consequences, she told him what Paul Miller had reported to her about Tommy.

Frank pressed his lips into the sort of amused half-smile that dismissed the whole business as simply crazy. "Tom—a mad-dog killer?" he burst out. "C'mon, Carol, how can you even worry about it?"

"It's been very unpleasant dealing with this man. I've been . . . rattled."

"What's Tom's reaction to this nut?"

Carol bit her lip. "Look, Frank, I haven't been able to reach him and—"

"Oh, that's right, he's down in Washington doing a dog-and-pony show for some potential investors."

"And please," she went on quickly, "don't tell Tommy I've discussed this with you."

"Of course, I understand." Frank lifted his napkin from his lap and tossed it onto the table. "Take some advice from me, Carol. If this guy Miller comes around again and lays any crap on you about Tom being a murderer, tell him you'll sic the cops on him . . . no, you know what you do: tell him you'll call *me*, and I'll come over and beat the shit out of him myself."

She left Frank at the door to her building. Again he hinted for an invitation to come up, but he seemed to understand that with Miller's accusation weighing on her mind the circumstances were wrong for pursuing romance.

"Parcel in the mail room for you, Miss Warren," the doorman said as she came in.

Carol went into the small room off the lobby and saw a single package sitting on the table. She looked for an E. B. Fox label, thinking it might be books from Binny, but there was no return address at all.

The UPS stamp was dated yesterday, marked Washington, D.C. From Tommy? It was meticulously wrapped, Carol noticed immediately—brown kraft paper folded at the edges and sealed on all sides with masking tape. The second thing that drew her attention was the block printing, hand-lettering by someone obsessed with details.

She began tearing off the wrapping in the elevator. As the doors opened on her floor, she pulled out the contents—a book, a beautiful old volume of the *Mother Goose* stories with a hand-tinted dust jacket and a fine cloth binding.

Holding her keys, Carol turned the pages to the copyright notice. The book was a 1967 limited edition by the New York Graphic Society with tipped-in etchings by artists of the day and a frontispiece by Marc Chagall. Having occasionally bought rare books for her own collection, Carol guessed that this one was worth at least several hundred dollars. Who could have sent it? She searched for a card in the wrapping. But there was none.

She unlocked her door, hung up her coat, and went into the living room. As she flipped the pages of the book, a piece of plain white notepaper flew out and fell to the floor. She bent down for it. "I thought you might appreciate having this," it said in the same meticulous block-printing as on the outside, "With apologies." It was signed simply, "Paul."

What the hell . . . ? Carol dropped the note on her drawing board as if it were infected. The "Paul" had to be Miller. But as beautiful as the book was, and even as an apology, such a gift was more disturbing than welcome.

What kind of relationship did Paul Miller imagine they had?

As soon as she opened her eyes the next morning, Carol headed straight for the living room and looked around for the *Mother Goose*, unable to remember where she had put it down. She had awakened with the realization that the book might provide exactly what she needed—a clue, a link to Miller in which he gave away more of himself than he'd intended. A means for her to become the hunter, he the prey.

She strode around the edges of the room, scanned the drawing table, and then checked the small entrance foyer. But for a few minutes the book eluded her.

At last she found it in the kitchen, perched on top of the refrigerator. She had put it there, she guessed, when she went to turn on the dishwasher before going to bed. She spent a moment looking at the cover—a watercolor of the classic image of Mother Goose, a white-haired old woman in a red cloak with children clustered around her. Then she opened the book and at once saw something meaningful, a name penciled on the first blank flyleaf. Written, she thought, in the shaky, overly curved script that might belong to a child fresh from her first few classes in penmanship. The name was Suzanne Miller.

Suzanne with a z . . .

The request he had made at the bookstore rose instantly into her mind—the inscription.

Miller's daughter, granddaughter . . . wife? Carol weighed the possibilities. One thing she didn't have to wonder about was the circumstances under which a child would proudly claim ownership of the book. It had been a gift, no doubt—which almost certainly meant that, at the time, it had been new.

Riffling the pages, Carol saw that they were smudged here and there at the edges as though by a child's soiled fingers. Turning past the inner title page, Carol checked the copyright date again: 1967.

So the little girl who had written her name in this book—a present she might have received soon after starting to read—was now in her late twenties.

Suzanne-with-a-z was probably Paul Miller's daughter.

Carol drifted back to the living room. For a moment she was pleased with her success at using Miller's latest invasion of her life to turn the tables. But then dissatisfaction set in. So Miller had a daughter named Suzanne. Could that be any help in tracing him? Finding out who he was, what personal motives he might have, whom he really worked for . . . ?

She sat down and inspected the book again. Except for the smudging, the only other mark to be found was a very faint, faded purplish ring, as though made by the wet bottom of a glass. As she turned the last page, Carol felt deflated; her attempt at playing detective hadn't yielded much.

And then, inside the back cover at the lower edge, she saw a sticker of silver foil, no bigger than a large postage stamp, with the name and address of the store where the book had been purchased:

THE BOOKWORM
117 State St.
Stamford, CT.

She moved to the phone. After more than twenty years, would it still be there . . . ?

The information operator found a number for the bookstore, and Carol called immediately. The man who answered sounded friendly and cooperative. But when she began probing for information about sales and customers going back two decades, he was unable to help. The store had changed hands a couple of years ago, he explained; all the old records had been cleaned out.

"You might try the former owner, though," the man offered. "His name's George Lumley. We still hear from him now and then. He moved over to Washington Depot and opened another bookstore called Wordsong."

"Wordsong," Carol repeated, and then asked for a more exact address.

There was no need, the man told her. Washington Depot was such a small town that a name would suffice. "That's why Lumley moved up there," he added. "The old man likes peace and quiet, and it was getting too built up around here."

After the call, Carol hesitated before picking up the phone again. Could she really learn anything about Paul Miller this way? How could she expect anyone to remember selling a particular book twenty-odd years ago?

Yet what else did she have?

Connecticut information quickly provided a number. A woman answered the phone, chirping out the name of the store: "Wordsong." Told that Carol was trying to reach George Lumley, the woman replied he wasn't there. "Actually he won't be coming in this week."

"Can you give me his home number?" Carol asked.

"I'm afraid he can't be reached anywhere for a few days."

"It's very important that I talk to him. Even if he's out of town—"

"Please believe me," the woman said in a sympathetic tone, "this simply isn't a good time to get him. But can I help?"

"If you're Mrs. Lumley, then maybe—"

"Mrs. Lumley died last year."

"Oh, I'm sorry," Carol said. She felt so clumsy for the gaffe that she nearly cradled the receiver.

But she couldn't break the thread, no matter how slender. She hung up only after leaving her name and her own number, with a message for George Lumley to get back to her as soon as possible.

11 THE SUN, GLINTING THROUGH the trees beside Huntington Bay, became a hundred splinters of light that stabbed painfully at Carol's eyes as she turned her little Pontiac coupe into Lloyd's Neck Road. She flipped down the sun visor and continued along the street of big Victorian houses toward a gray one with white trim and a wide porch at the middle of the street—the house in which she had grown up.

Her eyes were shaded now from the sunlight, but in her mind there were still splinters—fragmented thoughts she couldn't assemble in any reasonable pattern. The disorder set off a rising panic as she came closer to the house. How could she face Tommy if she didn't have a handle on what she felt? When she saw his silver Nissan sports car standing in the driveway, the breath seemed to rush out of her. She pulled to a stop, turned off the motor, then sat quietly at the wheel hoping her pulse would slow down.

Of course, she reflected, it wasn't just facing Tommy that had thrown her off balance. There was the whole situation with their father, the reason Tommy and she had agreed weeks ago that they would have to talk to him together this Sunday. At the time they had been simply a sister and a brother uniting to solve a family problem. Now it was hard to walk in and greet Tommy as if they were merely allies dealing with their father's illness.

Ducking her head to peer through the windshield

at the old house, she surveyed the damage wrought by time—the flaking paint along the white railing of the porch, the cracked frames of the bay windows. How different it had been when they were growing up. Her father was a spit-and-polish type, never one to let a brass doorknob get the faintest film of tarnish. Now, everywhere, there were signs of neglect.

The moment of nostalgic reflection brought some calm. Carol checked herself quickly in the rearview mirror, brushed back her hair with her fingers, and got out of the car.

As she mounted the porch, she saw the curtains part in the living room's bay window and her father's face peek out. He looked at her without expression before the curtain fell back into place. Reaching the door, she turned the knob of the old-fashioned brass bell-ringer. He might have recognized her, but there was no telling whether he would open the door—or even tell anyone else to do it.

It was the nurse who came. "Hello, Miss Warren."

"Hi, Mrs. Briggs. How's everything?"

The nurse allowed a tight smile that told Carol that "everything" was not very good. "We're managing," she said.

A hefty middle-aged woman who had begun the job late last spring by appearing daily in starched white uniforms, Mrs. Briggs had since relaxed into wearing a rainbow of pastel slacks, usually topped off by a Hawaiian print blouse or some slogan-bearing sweatshirt probably received from a grandchild. Today, indeed, she had on a blue pullover with a phrase emblazoned in white across the chest: I OWE, I OWE, IT'S OFF TO WORK I GO.

"He's with your brother in the living room," she said, closing the door after Carol.

"Are they talking? I mean, Dad . . . what's he like today?"

"Didn't have a bit of trouble recognizing your

brother, if that's what you're worried about. He remembered you were coming, too. Must have told me two dozen times how much he was looking forward to it."

Looking forward, Carol mused ironically as she walked back across the polished oak floor of the gallery toward the living room. At least he could still look forward, could imagine a future in which there were no absolutes. It was in trying to look backward where the tragedy lay.

Mrs. Briggs had walked with her to the portal of the living room. "Do you need me?" she asked.

"No, thanks."

Just before the nurse went upstairs to her room, she said, "I hope it goes all right. It really shouldn't be put off much longer."

Carol nodded to the nurse, then worked a smile onto her face as she prepared to take the turn into the living room. But at that moment her father emerged through the portal. He was nicely dressed in gray flannel pants, a white shirt, and the dark blue cashmere cardigan she had given him last Christmas. With his straight gray hair neatly combed and cut, he appeared physically well, Carol thought. He looked just as he always had when he'd come home from the phone company, pick up the newspaper from the table near the door, and go into the living room to relax.

"Hi, Daddy." Carol embraced him, attentive to the way he hugged her back, registering the slackness in his arms as if it were some kind of clue to the progress of his disease.

"Good trip out, honey?" he said as they moved into the living room.

"Sure."

"I always worry about you and that car, you know. Thing's too damn old."

A wave of sorrow washed over Carol. Her sporty Sunbird was only last year's model, a gift to herself with money received for illustrating a series of bank advertisements. The car her father was worried about was the beat-up second-hand Ford she'd driven all through college—a car she hadn't owned for eleven years.

But all she said was, "Don't worry, Daddy, there's a few more miles in this one." She flashed a look at her brother, who was sitting on the sofa with an album of old family photographs open in front of him.

He smiled at her, a message of courage as well as a greeting. "Hey, Carrie," he asked brightly, "have you looked at these lately? They're a hoot. C'mon, Dad and I were just going through them."

Bless him, she thought, for his breezy manner, his cheery optimism. Getting out the pictures was just the right thing—prompting Dad's memory with images that might cut through the fog of the Alzheimer's. Perhaps that would allow him to hear what they had to say without feeling too defeated.

With relief Carol realized that she was responding normally to Tommy, and again she was ashamed: even to have suffered a moment's confusion, she decided, had been a form of betrayal. Difficult as it might be for him to hear about Miller, Carol was now impatient to correct the error of trust. But there were other matters to take care of first.

For a while they all sat on the couch and turned the pages of the album, chuckling over pictures of Carol in her tank suit on the high school swim team, and Tommy going off to his prom with a gang of kids in tuxedos and crinolined evening gowns, and Carol and Tommy building a snowman with their father in the backyard. Seemingly at random—but perhaps because Tommy had not wanted to challenge their father with retrieving the most difficult memories—they had been flipping the pages back to front, the pictures getting older and older as they went. At first Pete Warren had little difficulty recalling people and places; the few faces he couldn't identify seemed to be the usual long-forgotten friends who found their way into everybody's candid snapshots.

But Carol was shocked by the enormity of her father's lapse when they came to a photograph of Tommy in baby clothes—no more than a year old—sitting on the lap of Culley Nelson's wife, whom they had always called Aunt Sarah.

"My God," said Pete, leaning over to look more closely at the picture, "it still hurts to look at her . . . your mother was such a pretty woman." He glanced to Tommy and shook his head, as if sharing a condolence. Carol saw there were tears in her father's eyes.

She wondered whether it was worth correcting him, then decided that letting it go was surrendering too much too soon. "Daddy, isn't that Aunt Sarah?"

Her father turned to her. "Sarah," he repeated in a small, hollow voice.

Feeling a need for support, Carol glanced to Tommy. But he was still gazing at the picture, as though charmed by the memory of himself as an infant. Carol looked back to her father.

"You know," she went on, "Uncle Culley's wife."

And then the light came into his eyes. "Oh, yes," he said simply.

"How about some coffee?" Carol asked, signaling Tommy that they ought to move to the kitchen table—the traditional family forum for settling thorny issues.

They went to the kitchen and while Carol brewed coffee, attempted small talk. It was difficult. When Tommy described his new house, Pete said, "You don't need a new house, you've moved too many times already"—even though this was only the second home Tommy and Jill had owned. And when Carol expressed the hope that her father would spend a day with her in the city, he replied, "It's too late for that now, sweetheart"—so that she wasn't sure if he accepted how taxing and joyless a trip would be in his condition, or whether he'd misunderstood the invitation and simply meant it was too late to go today. In either case, it broke her heart.

When coffee was ready, Carol poured cups all around, then she and Tommy told their father what was on their minds. The house ought to be sold, and the money set aside to pay for keeping him someplace where he would receive special care.

He took it placidly, seemingly with full comprehension. "But why couldn't I stay here?" he asked. "Briggsy and I get along fine."

Carol and Tommy exchanged a glance. It was the nurse's declaration that she couldn't cope with Pete much longer that had brought them here.

"Daddy," Carol said. "I love you with all my heart. I don't want you to be unhappy, and I wish . . ." She couldn't finish. Of course they all wished he had not gotten sick.

Tommy took up the slack. "You know it has to be done sometime, Dad. And isn't it best to make these plans while it's something we can *all* decide together— while you can still take part? There are good places to go, places you'll be comfortable, and have company—"

"And what if I won't go?" Pete shouted. "What if I damn well won't let you throw me away?"

Tommy extended his arm across the table and clasped his father's hand. "It isn't like that, Dad. You know it isn't. We just want to do the best thing."

Pete snatched up his coffee for a sip. But as he looked into his cup, his shoulders slumped, and then a pitiful burst of sobs escaped his lips.

Carol had never seen her father collapse so completely. The shock of it immobilized her, but Tommy rushed around the table and gently took the coffee cup from Pete's shaking hand. Then he knelt and embraced him, his large strong hands steadying the older man's heaving back in the same reassuring caress a parent would bestow on a child.

In a minute Mrs. Briggs appeared, drawn by Pete's moaning cries. With one look she perceived that the business of the day had been transacted.

"C'mon, Pete," she said firmly. "Time you had a nap."

Obediently he eased from Tommy's grasp. "Briggsy," he could be heard saying as he followed her toward the stairs, "you are one hard-assed woman."

"Guess it's settled," Tommy said quietly when they were alone.

Carol nodded. One thing was settled, anyway. She picked up a cup in each hand and carried them to the sink. Tommy followed with the third cup. She washed and he dried. Avoiding the matter on her mind, Carol talked about her date with Frank, telling Tommy how much she had liked him.

"Hey, look at that!" Tommy broke in abruptly. "A piece of that damn thing is still up there."

Looking up from the sink, Carol saw that he was gazing through the window at the big oak tree in an overgrown corner of the large backyard. Half stripped of its dying leaves, the skeleton of one large overhanging branch was revealed. And there, in a crook at the middle, the dangling remains of a thick loop of rope danced in the wind coming in off the bay.

She smiled at the memories it brought as Tommy unlocked the door leading to the yard and went out, down the rear steps. While she finished rinsing the coffeepot, Carol watched through the window as he walked across the garden toward the oak.

In a minute she went out to join him. The air was mild, perfumed by the tangy autumn smell of leaves burning down the block.

"We had fun, eh?" he said as she caught up to him.

They put their arms around each other and headed

toward the oak in the corner. "We had fun," she affirmed.

"And time marches on. There really isn't any choice but to sell."

"Maybe a family will buy it," she said. "They can clean it up, and the kids'll have a garden like we—"

"Kingdom," Tommy put in. "We called it our magic *kingdom*, remember?" They reached the base of the oak and Tommy pointed up at the branch where the rotted tail of rope was hanging. "And you'd be up there, stranded in the castle—"

"And you'd climb up and rescue me," Carol chimed in, clasping her hands together imploringly like the waif in some silent movie.

They laughed and remained for another few seconds, looking up. As clearly as if it were yesterday, Carol could remember her brother, just a boy, straddled over the branch tying on the rope—so worried it might not hold that he had tied one knot over another until there was a massive tangled clump that never had given way.

If only the link between them would prove so strong now.

She pulled away so that she could face him squarely. "Tommy, there's something I have to tell you, but . . ."

Reading her distress, he frowned with concern. "Don't hold back on me. If it's anything you need . . . you know I've got enough money now—"

"No, it's nothing like that." Carol rubbed her hands together and shivered slightly. The air was turning cold.

"Want to go in?" Tommy asked.

"No, not yet." Struggling for warmth, she hunched her shoulders up and pushed her hands down into the pockets of her skirt. She chose her words carefully. "A few weeks ago, a man started following me. Well, not exactly following, just . . . looking for chances to talk to me. What he really wanted, it turned out, was to talk to me about you." She saw Tommy stiffen—a sign of protective concern for her, she thought. "His name's Paul Miller, and he—"

She got no farther before Tommy exploded. "That goddamn maniac! He came to you?"

Before she could add a word, Tommy whirled, then took a step toward the tree and in a fury of frustration, pounded a fist against the trunk. "I could kill that crazy sonofabitch! Dragging *you* into his half-assed bullshit investigation."

Carol experienced a curious mingling of relief and anxiety. "Then you know all about it—this man Miller, the things he's saying."

"Do I ever! He's been to see me twice already."

Carol shook her head, perplexed. "But you never said a thing."

"Oh, and that surprises you?" Tommy crossed to her and went on in a sardonic tone. "A man calls for an appointment, walks in and tells me he's trying to find a guy who's killed I-don't-know-how-many women—forty, fifty? And then for the punch line he says I'm on his list of suspects." Tommy leaned down and his voice took on a scathing edge. "What the hell do you think I should do when he leaves? Call up all my friends—call my little sister—and pass it off as an interesting anecdote? 'Hey, you'll never believe what happened to me? Some jerk popped up in my life and accused me of being the bloodiest beast since Adolf Eichmann.' " He turned and looked despairingly toward the darkening sky.

"But if there's nothing to it—"

Again she had barely gotten out the words before he was ranting at her. "*If*? Can I believe my ears? Did I hear you say *if*?"

"Oh, Tommy," she pleaded, "you know I didn't mean it that way. I know there's nothing to it. I just meant . . . you've got to be able to stand up to it, treat it as if it's nothing more than a mistake, and then it'll be all right."

He gave her the same sort of forbearing look from times long past when he would treat her as his "kid sister"—who didn't know anything about tuning car engines or scoring football games or drinking beer. "Carrie, I wish it were that simple. I've sure as hell tried to keep it in perspective. First time this guy Miller turned up, I answered his questions politely, told him whatever I could. I thought that was that. But then a couple of weeks later, there he was again, walking up to me when I left work one night. This time he said his list of suspects had dropped from something like seventy down to sixty-five, but that I was still on it. Well, that made it a little harder to keep my sense of humor." Tommy's expression hardened. "And then I realized there was nothing I could do or say to satisfy Mr. Miller, because he's so revved up on this thing he can't let go. Did he tell you he's doing it on his own— that he isn't even a policeman?"

"He told me," Carol said. "But he didn't really explain how he got into it."

"To me either. There's something weird about it." Tommy inhaled deeply and let the air out in a sigh. "Unfortunately, that doesn't help me. He's already managed to make a little trouble between us, hasn't he?"

"I don't think so," Carol said. "We're able to talk about it, we trust each other."

Tommy smiled. "But it took you a while to get around to it."

"It isn't that I doubted you. I was just . . . mixed up."

"I have trouble myself knowing how to handle it. I get the feeling that the harder I fight to defend myself, the guiltier I'll seem."

Carol shook her head sympathetically. After a pause she said, "There's one more thing. I hope it won't create any extra problem, but, well, when my head was

spinning about this . . . I told Frank. We were out together, I was in the market for a sounding board." She
glanced back at Tommy. "Of course, he stuck up for
you."

Tommy stared at her for a second, then shrugged
and the shadow of hurt faded from his eyes. "Forget
it. You needed a sympathetic ear and I just didn't seem
like the best bet."

"Forgive me?"

"Sure." They started ambling back toward the
house. "Why shouldn't I? But that's what's so terrifying about Miller making his rounds with his goddamn
list—even my friends, who know me and trust me,
they're bound to have a moment of uncertainty. So
what does it do to other people? I'm trying to build
a business, Carrie, and that means going to banks,
dealing with guys who won't invest a dime unless they
know their money is protected ninety ways. Let them
think for a minute that I might get bad publicity—even
if I'll come out clean in the end—and it'll set me way
back. Maybe enough to kill the company."

"Oh, God, Tommy. I never thought of that."

"But how do I stop it? If I cry foul, it just looks to
Miller like he's struck a nerve."

They were nearing the steps into the house. "So
what will you do?" Carol asked.

Tommy sighed. "What *can* I do? Wait it out, I guess.
And hope that Miller crawls back into the same hole
he came from." Carol was about to climb the steps
when Tommy took her arm and held her back. "Whatever happens, though, I don't want you upset any
more. If that bastard bothers you again, let me know
and I'll set him straight. I'll sue him, I'll call the cops."

She put a hand to his face. "Let it pass. No matter
how many times Miller comes around, the people who
love you will be on your side."

"Christ, I'd like to believe that." He turned and continued climbing the steps.

Carol thought she heard a sadness in his voice. "Has Jill had any trouble with this?"

Tommy stopped, his head bowed. "I didn't know how to tell her, either."

For a second Carol was surprised that Tommy hadn't shared the problem with his wife—but only for a second. It was one thing to say you were suspected of murder; a friend could be found dead in a doorway and there was no shame in having to produce an alibi. But being on a list of suspects like Miller's, that was enough to bring you down in the eyes of everyone who knew you.

Yet Carol was sure that the wedge it would drive between her brother and his wife would be even greater if Jill found out from anyone but him.

"Tommy, you've got to talk to her. It'll be so much worse if you let it go any longer. I mean, if this man Miller isn't stopped . . ."

He had remained standing with his back to her. "You're right. It'd be hell if she heard about it from him. I'll tell her tonight." He went up the next step.

Carol caught him, put her hand on his shoulder. "Tommy. Anything I can do, you know—"

He laid his hand over hers. "Sure I do. You're the best." On the verge of preceding her into the house, he shook his head irritably. "Christ," he said, "what the hell did I do to deserve a problem like this . . . ?"

12 *STAY AWAY OR I'LL CHOP YOU DOWN*, Dana cried, *you're only a tree, you can't scare me.* The magic ax dropped into Dana's hand, and the forest of grasping trees around her retreated. Carol stretched and propped her new drawings against the lamp. Finally she was having a productive day.

The phone rang and she listened to her own voice on the answering machine. The beep came, and then:

"Miss Warren, this is George Lumley, from the Wordsong store in Washington Depot. I'm returning your call from last week. You can reach me today at—"

Carol ran to the phone and picked up. "Mr. Lumley, thank you for calling back."

"Oh, you're there," he said. "I've been away on business or I'd have been back to you sooner. I assume you're the same Carol Warren who writes books for children."

"Yes, I am," Carol said, pleased.

"My, what a delight to talk with you. I remember your first book so well—*Tiger, Tiger*, wasn't it?"

No matter how often she received praise, it always warmed her. But how surprising that George Lumley should recall a book published nine years ago, one that had sold only a few thousand copies. "I'm flattered that it made an impression on you," she said.

"We must've sold dozens," Lumley replied. "You know us booksellers, when we find a good book, we recommend it to all our customers."

"Honestly, Mr. Lumley, you don't have to—"

"Don't be too modest, Miss Warren," Lumley said with an amiable sternness. "Well now, what can I do for you? Locate an out-of-print book, perhaps?"

"Actually, it's a person, not a book, I'm trying to locate." She explained that she'd received a rare edition of *Mother Goose* with the Bookworm foil sticker and asked if it might be possible to trace the person who'd bought it.

"Goodness, that's a tall order," Lumley said. "We used those stickers back in the sixties, and we wouldn't have sales records that old. I don't think I could be much help."

Carol sighed audibly, but then another thought occurred to her. "Does the name Paul Miller mean anything to you?"

"Paul Miller? No. . . ."

"What about Suzanne Miller?"

Lumley repeated the name, again came up with nothing. "I could check some of our old mail-order records. Or maybe seeing the book would jog my memory. I don't know if it's worth your time, but maybe you'd like to bring it up here. I'd enjoy meeting you, anyway."

Carol leapt at the offer. She took down directions and made an appointment to visit Lumley the following afternoon.

The village of Washington Depot lay hidden off the highway in one of the tonier areas of the Connecticut River valley. It was two o'clock when Carol arrived at George Lumley's house, a classic colonial on a tree-shaded acre just off Main Street at the edge of town. Before she had reached the door, it opened to reveal a tall, elderly man with wire-rim glasses resting on top of his head in a mound of thatched gray hair. From his heavily lined, sunburned face Lumley seemed to be in his early seventies, but he had the broad chest and erect posture of someone many years younger.

"So you found me," he said, extending a hand. "I hope you left crumbs to find the way home," he added with a mischievous wink.

"I didn't know a witch was waiting for me," Carol said, smiling as she stepped over the threshold.

"You're in witch country," Lumley replied. "They used to burn them around here."

He led her to a low-ceilinged but spacious living room filled with country antiques, quilts, and bookshelves lining the walls. A pot of tea was on a low oak trestle table, and as soon as they sat down, George Lumley poured her a cup. Along with his late wife, he said, he had been in the book business for almost thirty years—first in Stamford and now here in Washington Depot.

"I dug out my grandson's copy of *With the Night Creatures,*" Lumley said, picking up a worn edition of Carol's book from the end table. "My grandson fell in love with Dana. Did you know that Charles Dickens said Little Red Riding Hood was his first love, that if he could have married her he was sure he would have known perfect bliss? That's the impact a fairy tale can have on a budding creative genius. That's why your work is truly important."

Carol smiled modestly. "If I started thinking of myself as important," she said, "I'm afraid I'd stifle the magic that makes the work happen."

Lumley fumbled through a pile of other books and held up a copy of Bruno Bettelheim's *The Uses of Enchantment,* the psychologist's exploration of the effect of fantasy stories on children. "Have you read this?" Lumley asked.

Carol shook her head.

"It's remarkable. I think that Dickens story about Little Red Riding Hood is in here. Bettelheim says that imaginary monsters, like the ones you create, have a crucial effect on the development of children. They help the little ones cope with their fears, prepare them to accept that there can be a dark side to human nature—anger and hatred and violence."

Lumley was a true book person, Carol thought, and indeed she did feel a moral responsibility to children. But she had not come all this way to discuss her work. She humored Lumley, talking for several minutes about how she developed her characters and stories. At last she lifted from her tote bag the edition of *Mother Goose* Paul Miller had sent her.

"That's the book, is it?" Lumley asked. "Let's have a look." He took it from Carol's hands and opened to the back flyleaf, carefully peeling the old pages apart. "Yes, that's our old sticker," he said wistfully. He turned to the front page and stopped at the flyleaf, his eyes resting on the inscribed name.

Carol waited, hoping something would connect.

"When you called," Lumley went on, "I thought you meant the wife's name." He ran his finger over the edges of the pages. "Suzanne," he read the name aloud. "You know, now that I'm holding this, I do think I recall them. A big family, three boys and the one little girl—that would be Suzanne. You don't see many big families like that, so of course they made an impression, used to come in with their father." Lumley leaned his broad shoulders back on the couch. "Miller, that's right. He was always buying books for those little ones. Believed in that, you know . . . developing their minds."

"Do you remember anything else?"

Lumley's eyes narrowed as he seemed to search his memory for a visual snapshot. "Let's see. A big fella, tall. Had a stodgy air about him, very formal and serious. Now, what makes me think that?" He put a hand to his cheek and stared up at the ceiling. "He always wore a hat, not too many men did that. The kind *my* father wore, old-fashioned, with the wide brim, you know, and a dent on top right down the middle . . . what do you call it?"

"A homburg," Carol said.

"That's right. Hardly anybody wears them now." Lumley put the book aside and stood up. "I'll get some fresh water for the tea." He crossed the room, but as he pushed through a swinging door into the kitchen, he turned and called out, "I forgot to ask you. Why are you looking for Mr. Miller?"

Carol had hoped Lumley wouldn't ask, and when the door closed she stood to look at the rows of bookcases. If she remarked on his collection as soon as he returned, maybe he wouldn't pursue his question. To judge from the books, he had wider interests than one would expect of a retired bookseller. Volumes on military history and the intelligence services filled nearly half of one wall, with an entire section devoted to the Korean War. Strange that a man so knowledgeable about children's books gave equal time to military history and tactics.

Lumley returned with the teapot.

"I see you're interested in the Korean War," Carol said.

"I served there. And it paid for my first bookstore."

Carol gave him a quizzical look.

"I retired from the Army at forty-two with a military pension. Otherwise, how could I have afforded a business as iffy as books? The way you young people look at it, I suppose you could say the defense budget did something good for a change." He stopped abruptly. "But where were we?"

Carol sat opposite him again. "You were trying to remember anything else about Paul Miller."

Lumley pondered a moment. "Can't dredge up another thing. I think we lost the family as customers even before we sold the Stamford store. They moved away, I think."

Carol started wrapping the brown paper around the *Mother Goose*. "That's all, then," she said, standing. "I appreciate your help."

Lumley rose. "You're very welcome. But before you go, I hope you'll leave some autographs with me." He brought out a stack of her books, one copy of each. "Sign them to William, will you? My grandson will treasure them."

Carol took the books and started to write, then noticed that except for *Tiger, Tiger* they were all fairly recent editions, hardly opened. "These are new," she said.

"I went right down to the store and got them the minute you said you were coming."

Carol smiled as she continued signing. Perhaps the bookseller could have told her about Paul Miller over the phone but had encouraged her to visit because he liked collecting autographs.

13 THE NEXT WEEK PASSED PEACEFULLY. Nothing had been settled, yet Carol felt decidedly better. On Tuesday morning Binny Madison called to report that *In the Dragon's Cave* had been nominated for the librarians' Bookmark Award; in a month there would a dinner at which the winners were announced. To celebrate the nomination Carol took in the Nevelson show at the Guggenheim with Margot, who was also buoyed by good news—with two job offers on the horizon, Larry was in better spirits, and so were the kids. Hearing about the nomination and the change in Margot's life seemed parts of a singular omen, a sign of bad times passing.

Then, after returning from a trip to the post office late Wednesday afternoon, Carol sat down at the drawing table to assess her day's work—and bucked backward on her stool. Her blue porcelain jar of brushes, with CAROL stenciled in white script, had been moved. Usually it sat on the right corner of her drawing table . . . and now it was in the middle.

Or had the jar really been moved? Maybe she had slid it over herself.

She searched through the apartment and found nothing missing. Was her imagination playing tricks? Calmer, she returned to her drawing board, flipped through her sketches . . . and again she had a sense of being assaulted.

She stared at her most recent drawings of Dana, the series with the trees crowding in on her. In Dana's hand, in all of the pencil sketches, there had been an ax to threaten and chase away the tree monsters. But in the last drawing of the series the ax was missing . . . erased.

Carol felt as if she were losing her mind. Had she changed the drawing and then forgotten?

No, she was sure. Someone had been in the apartment. But who would break in to do such a thing?

It came over her then, not in words but as a visceral force: a feeling of being invaded. Raped.

She had an urge to call Eric, but what could she say—that a burglar had come into her apartment . . . and stolen nothing?

That night she had trouble sleeping, finally dozing off around two-thirty, but the sleep was fitful, and at four in the morning she awoke in a sweat, feeling the clamminess of the pillow on her face like a cold rag. It was another two hours before she could sleep again.

During the next few days a subliminal turmoil began to grow and overtake her. No matter where she went, strangers' faces carried a threat, a danger. If she heard footsteps behind her, she crossed the street. If anyone stopped and held her glance, she ran past them to the nearest store. At the Food Emporium, wheeling her cart past the deli department, she saw a man with a gray hat at the checkout counter and ran up to him, ready to condemn, shout that he had to leave her alone. But the hat wasn't a homburg, and the man wasn't Paul Miller.

She had lost all sense of balance. Maybe, she thought, she was merely spooked by the idea of a man out there who had wantonly killed dozens of women, sought out his victims on city streets, in parking lots, anywhere he could snare the trusting and the innocent. The feeling wouldn't leave her, and she remained convinced that Paul Miller lay in wait just around the next corner.

But of course he never did appear, never showed his face.

Yet she couldn't help thinking, couldn't but wonder . . . why had Miller dropped out of sight as quickly and unpredictably as he had first appeared?

On Saturday afternoon Carol was at work when she was jarred out of her concentration by the loud bell of the house phone.

"A Mr. Gaines to see you, Miss Warren," the doorman said.

"Send him up, please."

Eric . . . he'd said he would call. Why had he come without letting her know? She shed her paint-streaked smock, grabbed a striped blouse from her closet, and ran a brush through her hair.

The front bell sounded.

"Hi, Carol," Eric said as she opened the door, "sorry to barge in like this. I happened to be in the neighborhood and thought maybe . . ." He stopped, gave a soft laugh. "Hey, no, that's not true. I didn't happen to be here. I made a detour just to see you."

It took her a moment to get her bearings. This wasn't the same Eric. He was out of uniform today— not wearing a starched white shirt, rep tie, and dark suit, but tan corduroy slacks and a canary-yellow boat-neck over a tattersall shirt.

She let him in and eyed him as he went past her into the foyer.

"You're sure this is okay?" he asked. "I have the day off and was on my way home, so . . ."

"It's fine," Carol replied. "I have some coffee on, if you'd like some. Decaf, though."

"That'd be great." He trailed her into the kitchen and she felt him at her shoulders as she poured the two cups. Then she led him into the living room, where he stared at the piles of books and supplies and the drawings strewn across the window seat.

"Your place is really nice," he said. "I wondered how an artist lived."

"Not so different from anybody else, I suspect." What was he *doing* here? Investigating, after all—in disguise?

She lowered herself into the club chair and he took a spot opposite her on the couch. There was an awkward silence while they sat staring at each other.

"It's been sort of a bad day," Eric said finally. "I got the idea suddenly that seeing you might make it better."

"What made it bad?" Carol asked quietly.

Eric's eyes moved restlessly around the room, as though searching for anything to settle on besides her. "Would you like to go for a ride?" he asked abruptly. "Up to the park, maybe? Or how about the Cloisters?"

She hadn't been to the medieval museum in years. The day was sunny, and Eric was apparently very much in need of a confidante.

His car today wasn't what she had expected either, not the plain dark sedan, which of course belonged to the police department, but a vintage MG convertible with the interior flawlessly reupholstered, and a spanking new paint job in dark bottle-green. On the drive up the West Side Highway, Eric explained that ever since his junior year in high school he'd been buying and restoring old cars in his spare time. "For fun," he said, "and occasionally some profit."

Sensing the pride he took in his hobby, Carol remarked on the MG. "It's a beauty."

Eric grinned. "Yeah. This one I haven't been able to part with."

The more Eric spoke about himself, the more he broke the mold of Carol's preconceptions about policemen. At night he took courses in law and sociology at John Jay College of Criminal Justice, not only because it might help him gain promotions but also out of genuine curiosity. "I missed a lot back in school," he told her. "I was a wild kid. Now I'm trying to make up for it."

"How wild were you?" Carol asked with a laugh. "You didn't ever break the law, did you?"

He glanced at her and smiled. "Don't bet on it. Nothing serious, but like I said . . . I was on the wild side. Maybe I'm making up for that, too."

"You mean by being a policeman?"

"I suppose. I'm glad I can help make the system work." He paused. "I don't want to make it sound like a great mission, because of course the other reason I'm a cop is purely selfish: I couldn't think of anything more exciting to do." He paused before adding, "Maybe I shouldn't admit it . . . but, even with all the nasty things that are part of being a cop, sometimes it's a real high."

"Even what you're working on now?" Carol asked reprovingly. "That's a strange way to talk about it, Eric."

He glanced at her again, frowning this time. "I know. That was insensitive. But . . . I . . ." He hunched over the wheel, peering intently at the road.

"What?" she prompted.

"Look, I'm the kind of a guy who puts my cards on the table. So here goes. I really like you, Carol. But if it's going to have a future, you've got to see me warts and all. You ought to know that I like what I do. To be honest about it, my work gives me a real kick. In fact, I bucked for working homicide because there's no bigger kick than solving the most serious crime of all . . . murder. That's why when the chance came along to join a special group working on this serial case, I asked to be put on it. Because there hasn't been anything bigger in years. Do you understand?" He gave her an earnest glance.

"It's not easy," she replied. "I know that who you are isn't totally dependent on what you do, or what you've seen. But it is hard to understand that there's a part of you that . . . gets a kick, as you say, out of being involved with something so horrible."

Eric kept a silence for a minute, and she was afraid she had offended him. But then he started to talk, this time staying in neutral territory. He asked how she liked to spend her leisure time. Was she a Mets or a Yankees fan? What good movies had she seen recently?

They arrived at the Cloisters, a medieval monastery the Rockefeller family had paid to have brought from Europe and reconstructed brick by brick on a bluff overlooking the Hudson River. The Unicorn tapestry, its most famous artwork, had been an inspiration to Carol from when she had first seen it as a child. Standing before it, she told Eric that she was often aware of borrowing from the rich, dense style for her own drawings.

After touring the museum they bought two Pepsis and ambled outside, to the promontory that offered a view of the Palisades across the Hudson River. The trees on the riverbank were erupting in red and gold, and Eric stood wordlessly in contemplation.

Carol broke the silence. "You said you'd had a bad day. Anything you want to talk about?"

He turned to her. "It was something my kid said to me."

Again Carol was surprised by how inaccurately she had pigeonholed him. The life she had imagined for Eric contained no wife or child, only a round of noisy singles' bars, with pretty young women lusting for the handsome cop, who was naturally receptive. "I didn't know you were married," she said.

"I *was*," he replied. "Divorced three years ago."

"I'm sorry."

Eric smiled self-consciously. "Nothing to be sorry about . . . isn't that what they always say?"

"I've always heard divorce is difficult to go through."

Eric shrugged. "With Joan and me it wasn't an angry thing. We just looked at each other one morning and realized it had been a long time since we'd enjoyed being together. She didn't like my friends, or worrying when I wasn't home for dinner. I really can't blame her for looking elsewhere for a life. I was in narcotics then, doing lots of stakeouts and late-night raids. It's not easy being married to a cop. We're friendlier now than we were then."

Carol realized why Eric had so quickly, even clumsily, exposed his feelings about being a policeman. "How old is your son?" she asked.

Eric smiled. The fine lines around his eyes wrinkled and he seemed to age a few years. "Doug's eight." The smile faded. "I should tell you this thing he said this morning that really shook me. I took him shopping to buy a down jacket he's been needing since last winter, and after that we went for a milkshake. And while I was sitting with him, he asked me if . . . if his mother and I weren't together anymore because she was afraid of me." He paused, his face tightened in concentration. "I shouldn't have been so shocked, I suppose. Because I knew it was really my fault. I'd been to dinner over at Joan's place last week, and it was the day after we'd found another body—a really good-looking girl, she was nineteen or twenty and when you saw the pictures of the body . . ." He expelled a breath of disgust. "I'd been able to keep it out of my head, but it got to me, it was like something had been torn right out of my gut. So when I was there that night, Doug asked me what I'd been working on . . . and I lost control. It just poured out of me like I was throwing up. I said there was a man out there who killed women and did all kinds of awful things to them, used them and cut them up and . . . and I'd do anything to catch the guy." Eric shook his head. "Stupid, unfor-

givably dumb. A kid shouldn't hear that stuff. I give
Joan credit, she didn't chew me out in front of Doug,
but when I left the house, she came after me and really
let me have it. I knew she was right. That's why I was
so flattened by what Doug said today. Look at the connection he'd made—that maybe all women should be
afraid of men." He shook his head, scolding himself.
"What have I done to my kid?"

"You've shown him you're human, Eric, that's all.
I don't think you can permanently scar a child with one
bad story."

Eric gazed at her a second, then a faint smile
touched his lips. "Well, you're the expert on stories,
so maybe you're right."

"Your son will be okay, I'm sure. Because he asked
one question doesn't mean he can't find the right answers for himself."

Eric reached out and took her hand, then pressed
it gently between both of his. "Thanks, Carol," he
said. "I needed to hear that I wasn't a total screw-up,
and coming from you, I'm ready to believe it."

"Why?"

"You just seem like a good person," he said.

His plain expression of appreciation, no less heartfelt for being slightly corny, touched Carol deeply.
What a paradox Eric was, she thought, one moment
confessing to the high he got from dealing with murder, and then showing himself as so unabashedly sen-
timental.

As they strolled on through Fort Tryon Park, Eric kept
hold of her hand. Carol felt keenly aware of many
other couples around them—having picnics or just sitting among the trees reading and talking, sipping
wine—and she couldn't help wondering what it would
be like if she became seriously involved with a policeman. How could she adapt to someone who regularly
traveled in the dark underside of the city?

Or was that, after all, a facet of him that actually formed a bond? Didn't she travel through dark worlds in the fantasies she was moved to create for her books?

When Eric asked how she had become an illustrator and writer, she found herself opening up to him. The roots of her career, she admitted, probably went back to her childhood when—in fantasizing adventures for herself and then drawing them—she had found relief from the sadness and isolation caused by her mother's early death.

"That must really be hard," Eric said sympathetically, "losing your mother when you're so young. I guess your brother had a hard time with it, too."

"I suppose," Carol said. "But he didn't show it as much." And then she stopped and flicked a sidelong glance at Eric. Was the way Tommy had been introduced into the conversation merely accidental?

Eric kept walking along, looking around at the woods, not even aware of her glance. When she dropped the subject of Tommy, he didn't pursue it, talking instead about how nice it was that she had succeeded so well in a difficult career. The reference to Tommy, she decided, had been nothing more than an innocent expression of interest in her background.

Arriving at an isolated spot near the top of a knoll, Carol asked if they could rest before walking back down to the car. "I'm out of condition for hiking," she said, leaning against a tree. "I should get out more, I guess, but I'm usually tied to my drawing table."

"Maybe I could liberate you sometime," Eric said. Bracing himself with his arm against the tree, he stood in front of her. "Take you off for a weekend into the great outdoors, somewhere we could get our exercise together."

She smiled at his ingenuousness, appreciating the undertone. "I'd love to," she said.

He was encouraged enough to slowly lean closer and lightly put his lips to hers. Carol let her arms go around him, yet she was grateful when he didn't make the temperature rise, backing off after one short, soft kiss. He understood tenderness, she thought, and she liked him all the more for that.

Straightening, Eric looked around at the woods, the ground dappled with patches of sun penetrating the branches.

"It's a shame," he murmured finally.

"What?" Carol asked.

"It's so nice here—makes me think how good it feels to cut loose now and then from the noise and dirt . . . how nice it would be to get away into the country with you." He faced her again. "But it's also been spoiled for me. Because these days I can't look at this kind of scene without, sooner or later, thinking of . . . him, and what he does in places like this."

He held her gaze for only a second before glancing back to the woods. Carol studied his profile, trying to find some hint of guile in his expression. This time, his mention of a police matter that might relate to her brother didn't strike her as totally coincidental.

"I thought we were here because you wanted to spend time with me," she said, disappointment showing in her tone. "But there's more, isn't there, Eric?"

He looked around quickly. "More?"

"You want the lowdown. This is all part of the investigation, finding out what my life was like—because it was also Tommy's life, the life of someone who might have—"

"No, Carol," he said forcefully. "That never occurred to me."

"Then why did you bring up this damn case, ask me about Tommy?"

He shrugged. "I don't know, I'm sorry. I have to say this, though: it did bother me when you called. How could you possibly think your brother might be involved? I had to wonder. Were you holding anything back, some information—"

Carol threw her arms up as she exploded at him. "No, damn it, no! Don't you see what's happened? It's Miller. For chrissakes, it's so bad he's got you suspecting me!"

Even in her fury she saw a weariness falling on him, his shoulders sinking. "Carol, I don't doubt you, not now, but it was so off-the-wall that you should even ask about your brother. The kind of animal we're dealing with, I don't believe he could've come from the same world you were raised in, the same family."

Finding her composure again, Carol said quietly, "So you don't think I'm hiding anything."

"No," he answered flatly. "I don't think you are. And I don't think you could."

There was a silence. Carol became aware of the solemn whirring of insects, the chirp of birds, the sounds of the woods. Then a spasm tugged at her throat, tears burned at her eyes, and she felt him enveloping her in his arms, his hands wrapping tightly around her shoulders.

"It's okay," he said, his words reaching her through her choked tears, "it's going to be all right."

As the anger drained out of her, she wanted more than anything in the world to believe him.

They rode down the West Side Highway without talking, the wind rushing in through the loose flaps of the convertible roof. In a trance of exhaustion Carol gazed out at the river and—in the distance over the Jersey shore—a plume of rust-colored pollution rising from the horizon.

"I apologize," Eric said finally. "I wanted a nice day with you and I blew it. Maybe it isn't fair of me to see you now. I mean, bringing my work into your life. If you don't want me to call again, Carol, then I—"

"No. I do want to see you, Eric."

"Thanks. And I'll try not to—"

A loud buzzing sound cut him off. Eric swore under

his breath and reached across her to the glove compartment. In one gesture he popped it open, pulled out an oversize telephone receiver, and quickly raised its aerial.

"Gaines," he said into the phone. He listened a moment, sighed. "Where?" he asked. "How long ago?" Another moment passed, and he continued, "Okay, I'll be down there in twenty minutes."

He handed Carol the receiver and she replaced it in the glove compartment. "Police business," he said. "I have to go somewhere. I'll take you home first."

"What is it?" she asked impulsively.

He was driving faster. "Another body was found. I have to look over the reports."

She had a strong urge to stay close to him, especially now. "Take me with you," she said. "Please."

"Carol, you may think you want to see this, but believe me—"

"Eric, you've told me how important your work is to you. Maybe you shouldn't try to cut everyone out of that."

But was it really because she wanted to understand Eric better, she asked herself as the car raced along . . . or was there something else she was desperate to understand?

14 THE LETTERING ON THE TRANSLU-
CENT GLASS PANEL, on the twenty-third
floor of the downtown Federal Office Building, read INTERSTATE LIAISON TASK FORCE. Eric
opened the door and held it for Carol.

In the center of a long, wide room were two rows
of scratched metal desks, twenty or so. The New York
City police, Eric explained, had joined several state
police divisions and the Justice Department in assem-
bling a group to deal with the problem of serial killers.
The investigators, five or six women among them,
were busy talking on phones or sifting through computer printouts. The place had a makeshift air, Carol
thought—with a Mr. Coffee machine on a low wooden
stand, a poster for Clint Eastwood's *Tightrope* tacked
on the wall, and blinking computer terminals set up
on cheap folding tables.

As Carol accompanied Eric to the rear of the large
office, several of the men and women lifted their heads
and nodded or gave a slight wave of the hand. "These
are the finest detectives in America," he remarked.
"Volunteers, like me. They put in for this case because
it's the most important thing going."

"But is this all you have—these people and a few
computers?"

"Unfortunately, serial killers just aren't a law-
enforcement priority. Seven or eight years ago we
hadn't even heard of serial murder, but now it's an epi-
demic. Some professor in South Carolina took all the

murder and missing persons statistics, fiddled around on a computer, and said there's probably five thousand victims a year nobody finds. Just picked off the streets at random . . . and killed."

Carol shook her head incredulously. The number of killers, their victims—the data seemed so technical, businesslike.

At the back of the large room they entered a narrow corridor. A tall, lean filament of a man in shirtsleeves was coming toward them. With curly white hair cropped so short his scalp showed through and webs of wrinkles around his puffy eyes, he had the appearance of an overworked high school principal.

"Hey, El," Eric greeted him, "how's it goin'?"

"Middlin' to maudlin'," he said.

Eric introduced him to Carol as Elward Daley, a retired FBI agent from Atlanta who was the head of the group.

"Pleased to meet you, ma'am," Daley said genially. "I'm real sorry to interrupt your day. But if you wouldn't mind, I'd much appreciate your letting me have Detective Gaines for half an hour, and then y'all can be on your way."

"Could I listen in?" Carol asked. Too late she caught Eric's dubious glance.

"Ma'am," Daley said, "I don't mean to be inhospitable, but it'd be best if you let me have Detective Gaines to myself. Meantime, we'll set you up with a cup of stale coffee and a dry cheese Danish." Daley let out a chuckle.

Eric led Carol to the end of the corridor and gestured into a lounge where there was a coffee maker, a soup vending machine, and a tray of sweet rolls. Carol tried one of the Danishes, but they were as awful as advertised. Restless, she wandered across the hall to a large empty room where the walls were covered in brown cork. Maps of Connecticut, New York, New Jersey, and Pennsylvania had been tacked up, and across the top of each were small photos of women aligned in rows, with strands of red thread running to red *x*'s on the maps. From the shape and style of the pictures, they seemed to have been cut from high school yearbooks. As her eyes moved across them, Carol was struck by how similar the girls looked . . . the pretty faces with big eyes, the long flowing hair, the bright smiles.

Victims, she realized. All dead.

For the briefest second she held her composure, and then she registered the sheer horror of it. In the next instant one face leapt out at her . . . Anne—in the photograph from the freshman book in college. Carol's eyes switched to the hand-lettered labels accompanying each strand of thread—a date, a place, a time, a file number.

As she scanned the labels, she heard voices and realized that Eric and Elward Daley were in an adjoining room.

". . . fits the MO down to the letter," the older detective said. "Late at night, trusting type, hidden good enough to decompose, it's comin' up on four months."

"And not a fiber or a tire track," came Eric's voice.

"Zero," was the drawled reply. "Woodsie is stayin' true to form."

Woodsie? Miller had called the murderer the Deep Woods Killer, Carol recalled. "Woodsie" was obviously a form of gallows humor.

To the side of the map room, a narrow portal led into a windowless cubicle. Carol went through and saw that photos covered the walls here, too. These, however, were glossy eight-by-tens, all in color, of wooded scenes, patches of leaf-covered ground, fallen branches . . . and in some, Carol saw, twisted bodies.

She had thought she was prepared. Maybe if she hadn't seen Anne's face, it would have been less gruesome. Or she could have performed the magic that enabled her to turn her dread into fantasies for children.

But this dread clung to her like a cloak of ice. "Oh, Jesus . . ."

Eric and Elward Daley came into the room. Eric stared at her as though puzzled by her prowling.

"Carol, you shouldn't—"

"Ma'am, you ought not to be here," said Elward Daley.

But Carol went on moving slowly closer to the wall.

"Carol . . . don't."

"Ma'am, I'll have to insist . . ."

The voices sounded to her like faraway echoes. In the picture before her, on a verdant thicket at the bottom of a hill, lay a skeleton, arms at its sides, the joints in the legs bent as though to remind her that they had once moved, once run . . . run, Carol thought, from whoever had done this. She took in the face, its sunken, rotting eyes fixed straight ahead and crying out *help me, help me.*

She spun, slammed into Eric, and threw herself past him, racing to the next room for light, for air.

The soup from the vending machine made her feel better.

Elward Daley's office had been spruced up with furniture that must once have been in someone's apartment—a wing chair and a tuxedo sofa in matching rose chintz. Eric sat next to her on the couch.

"How can anyone do that?" she asked, as much of herself as of Eric.

In a soft voice Eric said, "I ask the same question all the time. I hate to say it, but I don't think there are any answers." He paused. "Let me tell you about Alex John Bell. If you met Alex, you'd probably like him. A good-looking guy, pro basketball draft choice . . . the kind of boy who makes his parents proud. Sweet, lovable Alex killed seventeen women. There's George

Stano—he got convicted of nine murders in Florida, but they think he did at least thirty. And then there was Ted Bundy, a clean-cut all-American type who killed so many women they can't even be counted. And in five or six states. But catch this: he had a medal from the Seattle Police Department for capturing a purse snatcher. And he once saved a three-year-old from drowning. And he used to spend his spare evenings working on a suicide hot line—persuading people who wanted to kill themselves not to do it, not to throw their lives away. But he might go off right after doing that and kill one or two young women."

Carol held up her hand to stop him, shaking it back and forth as though to clear the air. "I don't get it. I know these men are careful, but they're crazy, too, so they have to make mistakes—"

"No," Eric interrupted, "it's not like that. You see, the ability to kill over and over means you can't have guilt, remorse. Or else you'd stop, or force somebody to stop you. But if you don't have guilt, then you don't want to be punished, and so you don't want to be caught."

"You will catch him, though," Carol said anxiously.

"Chances are," Eric said. "If we keep going long enough. But of course the longer we keep going . . ." He left the grisly truth unspoken. "There was a famous French criminologist named Locarde, lived in Paris in the late eighteen-hundreds, and he had a theory, he was the first one to lay it out, that every murderer leaves a signature at the scene of the crime. The murderer always leaves something, some piece of himself, no matter how small. That's at the heart of all police work, of every murder investigation we do, and it's always been true."

"So you'll find something," Carol said. "He'll leave a clue."

"No, this one may not," Eric said with a touch of despair, "may *never*. That's what so damned frustrating about serial killers. Locarde's theory doesn't apply to them. Maybe because this killer doesn't have a subconscious wish to be caught, he doesn't leave anything at the scene, not the slimmest link."

Carol found Eric's matter-of-fact tone unnerving. "You sound like you don't have a lot of hope."

"There is hope," Eric said. "But not in a clue from the killer. Someday there'll be a witness, or we'll have a license plate number or a make on a car. Or one of his intended victims will get away and give us a description."

"You have that woman who saw the crutches," Carol observed.

Eric nodded. "That was a break. Not much of one, but at least it's something." He gritted his teeth. "The hardest thing," he went on, emphasizing the words with a touch of fierceness, "is that the guy we're looking for probably seems normal. Maybe in all but the most crucial way, he *is* normal—which is why he can trap his victims." Eric stood. "I don't know why killers like this one exist, but I do know why he kills. It comes out of a need to exercise absolute control over people, to dominate them. He tortures and kills because it's the ultimate domination."

In Eric now, Carol heard a fever oddly like the one that drove Paul Miller. And then she thought back to Miller's describing how the murderer behaved, about his technique. Eric was doing it, too, talking as if *he* had stood at the killer's side.

Elward Daley appeared in the doorway of the office holding a light blue file folder in his hand. "Eric, can I see you for a second?"

Eric excused himself, leaving Carol to rerun her memory of the terrible photographs. In less than a minute he was back, standing in the doorway as he put the blue folder into his briefcase and snapped it shut. She perceived a change in him—an increase in the emotional temperature.

"Carol, I have to leave. Would you mind getting a taxi home?"

She stood up. "It's something new on the case, isn't it?"

"Please, don't ask me about it," he said. "C'mon, I'll take you down and help you get a cab."

She walked alongside him to the main part of the office. She heard a babble of voices rising from a group of investigators gathered around a single desk. But they fell silent as she came into the room.

Under their watchful eyes, she and Eric stepped into the hall. It was obvious that the task force's work had taken a major new direction, something to be kept confidential. In the elevator, then on the street, Eric kept a thoughtful silence. But after they had rounded a corner into a parking lot, he said, "I shouldn't tell you this, but I know it may ease your mind."

"Tell me what?" Carol pressed.

"We just got him," Eric said, a smile breaking across his face, "the Deep Woods Killer. In Syracuse. A bookkeeper who's been traveling around from job to job. After all this time, I don't even know what to feel. An end to this."

Until that moment Carol hadn't known the magnitude of the chaos Paul Miller had sown in her. Faltering for a moment, her chin sinking to her chest, she straightened up and tugged her arms around herself as though physically putting herself back together, healing wounds that had been inflicted over the past three weeks.

"I'm flying up there in an hour," Eric said.

Carol raised her eyes to him. "I always seem be thanking you," she said. "But thank you again."

"Maybe when I get back we can . . ." He shook his head helplessly. "Look, I have to go. We'll get together, okay?"

"That'd be fine," Carol said, though she didn't really know if it could be—how long it would take before she could relate to Eric without any vestige of the confused emotions that came from his being a policeman, and the suspicions that had hovered around Tommy.

He gave her a fleeting kiss, then dashed toward his car.

She stood at the edge of the parking lot, watching Eric's car until it turned onto Duane Street, then went to hail a cab. But as she raised her hand, the rage broke through, snapping inside her like the crack of a whip.

No, things couldn't be fine, not entirely. Because there was the matter of vengeance, long-simmering in her and now erupting to full boil. Paul Miller must be made to pay for the emotions he had unleashed in her. As she rode uptown, Carol found herself hungering for a chance to collect the debt due to her and Tommy.

15 LIFTING HER EYES FROM THE BOOK as she read aloud the last lines of *Dana's Dark Ocean*—lines she knew by heart after doing so many of these readings—Carol was charmed by the sight of two dozen seven-year-olds staring at her, eyes wide with wonder, lips tucked absently between their teeth, small fists clamped against their cheeks. There was nothing that touched her so much as looking at the faces of children when they were engaged in listening to a story.

" 'Then, with a swoop of his long silver-and-green tail, the sea monster dove down into the sea. And the last thing Dana saw was the line of bubbles that floated up to the surface, one by one by one, until she realized that they were spelling out a word.' "

Carol turned the final illustration around so the children could see it. "And there are the bubbles on the sea," she said. "Can any of you read what they say?"

Several kids called it out in ragged unison: " 'Love.' "

"That's right." Carol closed the book. "So the monster may have looked mean and ugly, but he had a heart."

The teacher, a pretty young woman in a pale blue shirtwaist dress, stepped in front of the class and prompted the children into applause. Margot's younger boy, Adam, went on applauding by himself for several seconds after the others had stopped. Though readings were usually arranged for Carol by her publisher, she had done this one because Adam Jenner was in the class and Margot had asked. Margot had come, too, and as she stepped forward from the back of the room, she gave Carol a brisk thumbs-up.

The teacher told the children to start forming a line for the walk to the cafeteria. "Do you want to eat with us?" she asked Carol and Margot. "We're having Sloppy Joes today."

Carol smiled. "No, thanks, Mrs. Jenner and I are going to grab a bite outside."

The teacher thanked her again and led the class out.

"How was I?" Carol asked Margot as they took their coats from the hooks by the door.

"As *Variety* says, boffo. A couple of kids have been on the fence about having Adam to their birthday parties, but I'll bet this swung it his way." They turned through the door into the corridor.

Carol stopped with a sharp intake of breath. Paul Miller stood erect against the wall outside, his overcoat still buttoned and the homburg held at his waist in both hands. His pose seemed incongruously servile, the stance of a butler waiting for his employer.

With one look from Carol to Miller, Margot sized up the situation. "Is this him?" she asked in a combative tone.

Carol's attention was directed solely at Miller. "They caught him," she declared. "They've got the man they want. So leave me alone. Please, Mr. Miller . . . just leave me alone." She supposed he had come to express regrets for disturbing her with suspicions now proven false. But she was still too enraged to care about an apology. She especially hated the fact that his showing up here meant he had been dogging her steps. She started past him.

"I'm very sorry, Miss Warren," Miller said, taking a hand from his hat to catch at her arm. "It wasn't what it seemed."

"You want me to call a cop?" Margot said, her war-like tone escalating.

Brought up short by Miller's grasp, Carol turned to look at him. The note of genuine regret she heard in his voice softened her. She acknowledged Margot's question with a small shake of her head. "No," she said, "you don't call the police to deal with a sick man."

"Miss Warren, when I said I was sorry, I don't think you understood. I'm sorry it isn't over." His hand was still resting on her arm, but the touch had lightened. She made no attempt to wrest free. "That bookkeeper in Syracuse," Miller continued. "They let him go in twenty-four hours; he wasn't what he seemed. Not the man they want, but just one of those people looking for a moment in the spotlight, a man ready to confess to something he didn't do."

Carol stared at him, robbed of words. It wasn't only that he had brought news which—if it could be believed—meant that this ordeal with him would go on. She was equally stunned by his awareness of information that, as far as she knew, had yet to be made public—things Eric had told her in confidence.

"How did you know about that bookkeeper?" she demanded.

"Carol, honey," Margot urged, "let's get out of here. I think you're right, this man is sick."

Carol had changed her mind. She needed to know if Miller was telling the truth—and if, God forbid, he was, how he had even learned about the arrest upstate.

He had taken his hand off her arm. "I'll explain," he said. "But I want to talk to you alone." He glanced at Margot, attempted a cordial smile in spite of her own furious expression, then looked back to Carol. "If it's not convenient now, we can arrange it for later."

Carol glanced to Margot. "Could we skip lunch?"

"I don't mind. It's you I'm worried about. I think you shouldn't trust him."

"I don't," Carol said. "But I want his explanation."

Margot hesitated. "See you later, darlin'." She faced Miller, as if ready to issue a warning, but then turned and walked toward the stairs at the end of the hall.

"Do you want to talk here?" Miller said after Margot had gone. "Or shall we sit down?" He gestured into the classroom with its scaled-down chairs for children.

"There's a playground outside," Carol said. She was past caring whether or not she and Miller were alone. There had been enough of those occasions now, and whatever harm had been done, it had never been physical. But the world that Miller brought with him, dark and hateful, had a physical effect on her, made her feel closed in. She needed breathing space.

They went down the steps at the end of the hall and through a rear door to a large, fenced-in playground with a jungle gym at one corner and several wooden benches. No children were out, and the huge empty yard was bleak under the overcast November sky.

As soon as they settled on the nearest bench, Carol fired off a question. "If it's true that the man who confessed is innocent, then are you here because my brother is still a suspect?"

"Yes."

"And have you come," Carol said sharply, "just to let me know the screws are still on? Or because you think I'll tell you something that proves my brother is guilty?"

"I'm here because the case is still active," Miller said mildly, "and as long as it is, I'll keep talking to whoever might offer a chance of stopping the slaughter."

Carol held back the venom she felt. "Listen, Mr. Miller, I've spoken to my brother. I know you've seen him, and he's tried to deal with you openly and honestly. You ought to know by now that he couldn't possibly be the man you want."

"If this killer were a man who *looked* guilty, Carol, he'd have been stopped by now."

Carol turned away in exasperation. She was annoyed at his shift to a kind of intimacy—casually using her first name—but she let it go.

"Look, there are only a few things I'd like to ask you," Miller said.

Something was different. At first Carol couldn't put her finger on it, and then she realized suddenly that he had actually been ready to ask direct questions about Tommy, interrogate her as if trying to establish guilt, perhaps to break down an alibi. The switch from his past strategy, in which he'd always seemed to appear for no reason other than to put her off balance, somehow infuriated her.

"Damn it, you want answers, but you don't give any. Well, you're going to answer my questions *first* before I'll hear any more of your accusations against my brother."

"I've made no accusation," Miller corrected her. "I've only said he's one suspect among many."

"But what in hell makes you an authority?" Carol shouted, unable to contain herself now. "Who in God's name are you, Miller? How did you know about that bookkeeper in Syracuse? Where did you come from . . . and where do you go when you disappear?"

"You deserve answers to everything," Miller said evenly. "It's one of the reasons I wanted to see you." He paused and sat up, straightening his coat with a shrug of his shoulders as though neatening himself after a fall. Resuming, he didn't look at her but kept facing straight forward from the bench, looking off to a distant corner of the playground. "You know I work for myself, Carol. I get some cooperation from the authorities here and there—the police in many places have come to know me from my involvement with the case—but I have no official connection." Like a blind man listening for a voice, he leaned toward her slightly, but he anticipated the question without having it asked. "But why do I do it—you might want to

know—and how can I afford it? Because of course
there's no pay . . . it's just a labor of love." Miller
looked down at the ground as he went on. "I had a
business until three years ago—security consulting. I
provided advice to banks, racetracks, some defense in-
stallations, places that had something they didn't want
to lose—money or weapons or secrets. It was a very
good business. And then—"

There was a burst of raucous noise as a gaggle of
children suddenly tore into the yard for recess. Miller
glanced over at them, and Carol saw his face touched
by a smile so quick it was almost a twitch. As the children ran to a far corner of the yard and the noise
faded, he turned to her and asked absently, "Where
was I?"

"You had a business, and then . . ."

"Oh, yes . . . then." Abruptly he seemed to change
the subject. "I should mention I had a family, too.
Three sons and a daughter. I'd lost my wife when the
children were fairly young, so I brought them up alone
right through college."

Carol almost blurted that she knew about the children, but she stopped herself in time. He mustn't
know she had checked up on him.

"My being both mother *and* father to them, I think
that's important to having you understand why I do
this now. Why I never gave it a moment's thought almost from the day they found Suzanne."

No sooner was the name mentioned than Carol
thought she knew the rest of the story, but he had already continued.

"My daughter was twenty-four when she disappeared—a little more than three years ago. She was
a remarkable young woman, in her second year of
medical school at the University of Connecticut, and
one night she stayed late to make up some lab work.
There were witnesses who saw her in the laboratory
at around ten o'clock, and sometime after that she left

to walk back to her dormitory. She never got there."
A hoarseness had come into his voice, and he paused
to clear his throat. "She was found in the wooded hills
above the Connecticut River valley ten months later.
Her body . . ." His voice gave out. "Excuse me," he
said, almost in a whisper. He cleared his throat again,
and when he continued, this time the tone was
stronger, more resolute. "There are animals in those
forests—raccoons, foxes, even dogs set loose by bored
owners that turn wild, and of course they forage on
carrion—"

"Mr. Miller," Carol broke in, "I understand."

He swiveled his head slowly to look at her. "No,"
he said with a quiet ferocity. "You *think* you understand. But you can't, not until you see it."

"I've seen pictures."

"Pictures!" he roared, loud enough that it echoed
across the yard. Several children stopped and looked
at them, and Miller brought his voice down again. "I
was *there*, Carol, the police took me. And I saw nothing
but the skeleton of a dismembered body, bones
chewed and scattered by animals. And from the remnants of her clothes, and in the way certain objects lay
near her remains, things like a screwdriver, and a huge
rubber thing—a sort of makeshift dildo, if you know
what that is—the indications were very clear that my
daughter had been horribly tortured and sexually mu-
tilated." He bent close to her, his eyes burning. "And
the same thing," he added in a seething half-whisper,
"has been done to every single one of the victims."

Carol was mute with shock. The obscenity of what
she had heard was compounded, she felt, by hearing
these things even within sight of the children.

Miller took a deep breath and continued. "After the
police told me that Suzanne was only one of many victims of the same killer—the count was almost twenty
at the time—I knew what I had to do. I went home that
day and arranged to turn my business over to associ-

ates. I had money enough to live on for five or six years. I was sure that would give me time." He gave her a troubled glance. "The time's more than half gone."

Miller glanced away to where the children played, and Carol took the moment to study him, the rugged face that suggested an explorer—a man venturing into a hostile unknown—framed by the odd counterpoint of a hat one usually saw in pictures of diplomats from past eras.

"Mr. Miller," she said, "tell me—"

"Paul," he put in as his eyes came back to meet hers.

The invitation to join him in the intimacy of friendship—or the illusion of it—jarred Carol, and she tried to ignore it. "Why," she finished her question, "is Tommy on your list?"

He answered without hesitation. "Most of the reasons are purely circumstantial. The victims have all come from an area that takes in four states—New York, Connecticut, New Jersey, and Pennsylvania. In order to commit these murders and not arouse any suspicion, there's no doubt that the killer must live within a few hours' drive of the scene of every crime. So he's able to sleep in his own bed every night—or else to have good reasons, like traveling on business, for not being there. Do you follow me so far?"

Carol nodded passively. What Miller had said applied to Tommy, of course . . . but also to millions of other people.

"There's another similar aspect in quite a few of these crimes, cases where the victims were nurses or lady doctors or women visiting hospitals—and the point from which they disappeared was a hospital parking lot. And of course, your brother's business is involved with selling specialized equipment to hospitals . . . and so he'd have reason to be in the vicinity."

"But these things happened in particular places at

particular times," Carol observed. "Tommy should be able to satisfy you that he was somewhere else. He probably keeps records of his business trips."

"Yes, there are records," Miller agreed, "and I'm taking that into consideration. But you have to realize, Carol, that a guilty man would want to fudge that. What your brother has given me to look at—"

"So he willingly showed you his records."

"Some," Miller admitted. "But there's no proof that they were accurately kept."

"All right, Paul," Carol demanded, "what else?" The acceptance of familiarity slipped out, startling her especially because she was irritated with him. What hope was there to deal with him if he brushed aside even reasonable objections for the sake of clinging to his prejudice?

"Physical description," he replied quickly. "There are a few instances where witnesses recall seeing the victims talking to a man before they disappeared. Descriptions of that man—light brown hair, slim, tallish, good-looking—all bear some similarity to Tom."

"Good God!" Carol erupted. "Do you call that evidence?"

"I never pretended it was. It's only the background against which more significant information can be assessed. And there is one particular factor that weighs against your brother more heavily—something that makes him one of just fifty-one men who still can't be ruled out."

Fifty-one. Carol registered the number; the list was shrinking. "You mean that Tommy knew Anne Donaldson?"

"No. If anything that favors his *innocence*. Because this kind of random killer tries to avoid any ties to his victims. It's easier to stay in the clear that way."

"So that makes him innocent!" Carol said harshly. "Then what makes him guilty?"

"There's a case, up in Rowayton, Connecticut,

where a witness saw a victim get into a car with a man. When the police questioned this witness, she recalled some details about the car—that it was pale blue or gray; a compact sedan of Japanese make; and more to the point, she retained an impression of the license plate."

"An impression," Carol repeated dubiously. It was a strange word to use about something that ought to be an absolute.

"Specifically, she thought the registration was a combination of three digits and three letters—and most important, that two of the numbers were eights. That's enough to really narrow down the possibilities. A couple of the police departments involved in this case have done a computer search of the auto registration files using the information. That's what led me to your brother."

"He doesn't own a car like that," Carol protested. "And the police don't have him on their list."

"The company car your brother drives," Miller shot back, "is a gray Toyota sedan, registration 858-BFG."

Carol digested it all for a moment. Then she threw up her hands. "Two eights, for God's sake. Your one-and-only precious witness has an *impression* of a license with those two numbers in it . . . and from that my brother gets dropped into your hopper of bloodthirsty crazies. How can it come down to nothing but two lousy eights?"

"Because," Miller replied quietly, "there's so little else."

"It's simply not fair," Carol declared stridently.

"Nor is the killer, whoever he is. The women he's butchered are smart, some of them highly accomplished. Yet he gets them to go willingly. That means he's a genius at deception, Carol. It means," Miller added, "he can fool anyone."

She got the innuendo—that she could be fooled even by her own flesh and blood. "You're so goddamn sure you belong in this, aren't you, Paul. You've suffered horribly, I don't doubt that, and I'm sorry. But does that give you the right to make others suffer, people who are innocent? You've got your list of—how many, now?—fifty suspects, and you're going around asking questions, and so there are fifty men, and all the people who love them, suffering, being wounded in a way themselves . . . and yet maybe *all* of those fifty men are innocent?" Her voice never wavered, though tears were brimming in her eyes. "What gives you the right to do that when there are so many police and—"

"The police aren't equipped to deal with this," Miller announced, and the arrogance and bravado of it froze Carol's words. "Don't you see? Cases like this cover too many jurisdictions, get tangled up in the jealousies between police departments, lost in their internal competition. Then there's the sheer weight of all the information that has to be checked. Thousands of clues, so the most valuable one can get buried in the clutter, overlooked by some clerk who's thinking about last night's argument with his wife." Miller seized Carol's arm. "But that can't happen with me, Carol. Because this is my life. There's nothing else for me, nothing more important. Nothing! There never will be."

His grip tightened and she winced. When she turned to stare into his face, he withdrew his hand. But as she looked at him, Carol felt a perverse collision of emotions: fury and compassion, damnation and pity. He was a man obsessed with a mission that could only bring her increasing pain—at least until she could satisfy him of Tommy's innocence. Yet she felt a rush of forgiveness because she knew that, no matter what he did, his pain would always be greater.

"Questions," she said. "You said there were things you wanted to know. . . ."

He hesitated. He looked tired now, older, depleted by the ordeal she had put him through. "General things," he replied. "Whether he's ever seemed especially edgy or distracted . . . given you any reason to doubt—"

"Never," Carol said, not needing to hear the rest.

Miller spent another long, silent moment gazing at her. "Then I don't think there is anything else." He stood up and touched a hand to his homburg, that familiar, old-fashioned tip of his hat. "Thank you very much, Carol."

The abruptness of it left her off balance. She stood. "Will you . . . need to see me again?"

"That depends," he answered slowly. "Good-bye."

Automatically she echoed the word.

For another moment Miller kept his hazel eyes trained on her face. And then he stood, pulling himself up from the bench in what seemed an exhausting effort of will. Carol was half to her feet when he turned quickly and walked away.

It was curious, she thought as she watched him go. What had he thanked her for? She'd told him nothing. More than needing to ask questions, she felt, Paul Miller had come only to give her answers.

16 "YOU DON'T FIND UNUSUAL THINGS like this in the malls," Jill said, standing at the window of Charivari on Columbus Avenue. "It's why I love coming into the city to shop."

Carol's sister-in-law had called early in the day to suggest a shopping expedition. "I've always admired your taste, you know," she said. "You have a wonderful sense of color and fabric." But in Jill's voice Carol heard an overblown, too-cheerful gaiety, and an invitation out of the blue was not her style at all.

Carol could guess what was on her mind. Tommy had probably told her about Paul Miller. And yet during lunch at Tavern-on-the-Green and walking up Columbus Avenue, Jill had said nothing. While tempted to probe her mood, Carol nevertheless held her tongue. Maybe she had been wrong, after all. Maybe Jill had come only to shop.

In Charivari, a store with trendy clothes—leather-patched mesh jumpsuits and extravagant square-shouldered blouses—Jill selected dresses to try on. While she went to the dressing room, Carol sifted through mounds of Hungarian-made sweaters with exquisite detailing. She looked at a price tag: $420. Too expensive, she thought, but it was fun seeing how you could change your whole appearance with a single unique garment.

She had slipped in and out of several sweaters before realizing that Jill had been gone an extraordinarily long time. Carol walked to the rear of the store and

ducked her head into the curtained changing room.
The narrow latticed doors were all closed, and there
was no sight of her sister-in-law.

"Jill?" she called.

Carol called louder, and still there was no answer.
Had Jill returned to the front?

Then, from the last cubicle in the row, Carol heard
a faint keening—someone whimpering, she realized.
She moved to the door and peered through the slatted
panel.

"Jill . . . ?" Carol turned the knob, gently pushed
on the door. It opened a crack, and when there was
no resistance, she gave it a light shove.

She saw first a bare shoulder, an arm folded against
the wall. Then she took in the rest—the bra half-
undone, the bare breast pressed against the wall, and
the single eye visible, makeup starting to run beneath
it.

"Here, have some wine, you'll feel better."

Stretched out on Carol's couch, Jill waved the gob-
let away. "Do you have some herb tea?"

In the store Carol had held Jill until she stopped crying and had helped her get dressed. But Jill still had
been too upset to drive crosstown, and after urging
Carol into the driver's seat, she remained silent for the
entire ride except to mumble repeated apologies for
"ruining" the day.

Carol brought a cup of chamomile tea and a plate
of shortbread biscuits to the coffee table. "Jill, honey,
talk to me."

Jill sat up and purposefully straightened her shoulders. "I'm so sorry about all this. It's not like me. You
know I'm strong, Carol, but . . . oh, I wanted to believe
that things could go on . . . that everything would be
normal."

"Why shouldn't they?" Carol said, not wanting to
ask Jill directly what Tommy had told her.

"You don't have to play dumb, Carol," Jill said with an edge. "Tom said you know all about this person Miller—the charges he's making."

"Jill, there are no *charges* being made. There's an investigation—"

"And Tom's part of it!" Jill broke in tearily. She grabbed up the cup of tea but didn't drink from it, as if she simply needed something solid to hold on to. "I just don't know what to do, who to turn to. I almost called my parents, but I can't tell them, it would only worry them. I don't dare tell our friends, do I? I have exams coming up, Carol, papers due . . . but I can't concentrate at all with this dreadful thing hanging over me." She started to sob again, and in a matter of seconds it became a wail. "Oh God, oh God, why is this happening? Tell me *why*."

Carol soothed her until she was calmer, sharing an admission of her own loss of concentration in the wake of Miller's charges. "But listen, Jill. What keeps me going—what can help us all—is that I know we'll come out all right. Sooner or later we'll find out why Miller is after Tommy, and we'll put this behind us."

"Sooner or later," Jill echoed hopelessly. "But there isn't time if it's later."

"What do you mean?"

Jill looked toward the window, gazing at the distant skyline with an almost palpable melancholy. "I'm going to have a baby," she said. "The results came back yesterday."

Carol reached out impulsively and seized Jill's hands. "But that's wonderful. You've wanted this for so long."

Jill stared back at her, unmoved.

"Isn't Tommy thrilled about it?" Carol asked quickly.

Jill looked down and tugged her hands from Carol's grasp. "I haven't told him. All last night . . . I just couldn't."

"Oh, Jill," Carol said, sighing with frustration. "It's such good news, and if ever Tommy needed a lift—"

"But I *can't*," Jill shot back. "Not now. What if . . . what if the way things go . . . it turns out . . ." She shifted her eyes to look squarely at Carol. "I mean, if something horrible happens . . ."

Carol recoiled in her chair. "Jill, you can't imagine for even a second—"

"I can," Jill cried out shrilly. "I can imagine all *kinds* of things. What if this man Miller keeps chasing Tom? What if there's some circumstantial evidence and Tom can't prove he's *not* guilty? And what if Tom is accused publicly, if the newspapers print stories, if television cameras come to our house and—"

"Stop, Jill," Carol commanded. "None of that will happen."

"Are you so damned sure? He's under terrible pressure, Carol. You see, don't you—you see that if I told him about the baby now, he might . . ." She broke off.

"Might what?" Carol pressed.

"He might want me . . . not to have it. And the way I'm feeling . . . so confused about everything . . . I don't even know if I'd fight that. It might even be the right thing."

Carol stared in horror at her sister-in-law. "Right? How could that be right?"

Jill sat for a moment kneading her hands, her breathing irregular. She seemed on the verge of hysteria, and when she spoke again, her voice was low and raspy. "Carol, he's your brother, so please don't be angry with me, but I can't help it . . . he's my husband, and I love him . . . but I still can't help what's going through my head."

"No," Carol said softly, not waiting to hear the rest.

But Jill talked on. "I don't know if I could have the baby, if I think there's even the tiniest chance—"

"No!" Carol screamed. "You can't think that way, Jill. You'll poison your life. Listen to you, ready to give up something you've wanted, dreamed about for years. All because of a charge that's meaningless. Jill, I've talked to the police. Tommy is not a suspect."

Jill lifted her chin and eyed Carol warily. "Who in the police? Why would you talk to them?"

"Because I have a . . ." She paused, not certain how to describe Eric. "I have a friend who's a policeman. I met him at Anne Donaldson's funeral. He's working on these cases and he checked his files for me. Tommy's name has never even appeared."

Carol's reassurance was apparently the tonic her sister-in-law needed. Picking up her cup of tea, Jill sat back and let out a long breath of relief. "I needed to hear someone sensible," she said. "I almost called the psychiatrist I saw a couple of years ago, but I was afraid even to talk to him. It's like anything else, I guess . . . you keep things bottled up, they start to seem worse than they are. I probably haven't been very good for Tom these past few days."

"So go home and give him the good news. Get on with the important things. That's what I'm trying to do."

Jill agreed. She was supposed to meet Tommy for dinner tonight at a lovely country inn just north of Saddle River. As she mentioned it, her eyes took on a brightness that hadn't been there all day. She leaned forward and clasped Carol's hands. "It is good news, isn't it?" she said. "Next time maybe you and I can shop for things for the baby."

17 CAROL REACHED TOMMY in his office just
before lunch the next day. She had barely said
hello when he began to crow excitedly. Jill
had told him he was a father-to-be.

"I'm in heaven," he said.

"It's wonderful news," Carol said.

"I thought it would never happen."

"Why not?" Carol asked, surprised.

"We never said anything to you, but the doctors had
some doubts about whether Jill could get pregnant."
There was a pause. "I would've talked to you about
it, Carrie, but it made Jill uncomfortable—and we
were a little superstitious. Like Dad used to say, don't
borrow trouble."

Carol smiled. The phrase was their father's favorite
homily, almost an incantation. If you avoided thinking
about trouble, you wouldn't invite any.

"So how was Jill when you saw her yesterday?"
Tommy asked. "It's strange that she went to you to
talk about the pregnancy before telling me."

"She's upset, Tommy," Carol said sympathetically.
"Can you blame her?"

"No," he allowed, "who could? Did she seem okay
to you?"

Carol said that Jill was fine and had delayed breaking the news about the pregnancy only to avoid bur-
dening him at a pressured time.

"Thanks for taking care of her," Tommy said. "All
things considered, I guess she's handling this Miller

thing pretty well. But sometimes I look at her, Carrie . . . like last night at dinner. She had black rings under her eyes—she's not getting enough sleep. When I think about Miller, I want to get my hands around his neck and—" Tommy caught himself. "Uh-oh," he said with forced lightness. "I've got to be careful what I say, don't I?"

"Being angry sounds normal to me," Carol said encouragingly.

"To tell the truth," Tommy said, "I'm not sleeping so well either. You know me, I could snore through an atomic blast, but yesterday I was up at three in the morning. I went into the library and sat thinking until the sun came up. Carrie, there's a bad smell about all of this—something right in front of my eyes that would explain it but that I'm not seeing."

Carol said nothing for a moment, pained by her inability to soothe his anxiety. She admitted then that Paul Miller had talked to her again.

"Jesus, Carrie," he exclaimed furiously, "that's the end! I'm calling the cops—this minute. There's no guessing what this son of a bitch will do."

"Wait," Carol said. "It wasn't a mistake to talk to him." She told Tommy the reason for Miller's quest— the loss of his daughter—and the one other fact she had learned that might be useful: the coincidence of the license plates.

"Yeah, he told me that, too," Tommy said bitterly. "And the stuff about the cars and the description. But it's so crackpot, Carrie. Fifty victims, for chrissakes. When am I supposed to have *time* to kill all these people?"

Carol could sense now what Jill had implied. The strain on her brother was building; she worried that something in him might snap, and in a way that would make him look more unstable.

She heard his secretary's voice coming through an intercom in the background.

"I have to go," he said. "The foreman of our North Carolina plant is on the line. I'm still trying to run a business here. Do you know how crazy this is making me? Today I actually wondered if one of my competitors had stirred it up. Listen, thanks for calling."

"Bye," Carol said. "Feel better, it'll be okay."

"Thanks, I love you."

For a moment after hanging up, Carol found herself analyzing Tommy's mood as though every word were a hieroglyph. What did this phrase mean, or that one? If he were crazy, and a murderer, wouldn't he try to disguise his anger at Miller?

On the verge of standing to pace around the room, Carol stopped herself. Paul Miller was like a contagious disease, she thought. If you were exposed to his madness often enough, you caught it. And she was determined not to.

At around six the phone rang. She laid her chalk aside and answered.

"Carol, it's Frank Matheson. I just got in from Connecticut and thought you might like to join me for dinner. For you, I'd cook my most complicated specialty."

Carol was pleased to hear from him, and for a change she wanted company. "I'll bite," she said with a laugh, "no pun intended."

"It's a surprise, you'll have to rise to the bait."

She scribbled down his address and said she would be over in half an hour. After a quick shower she spent a few minutes putting on her face and slipped into a tan wool dress. In record time she was on Third Avenue hailing a cab.

Frank lived in a prewar building on West End Avenue, decorated with crenelated stone balconies and gargoyles on every cornice. The lobby had seen its glory days, but with marble walls and Deco sconces it still maintained a ghost of its grandeur.

In the elevator, after she told the attendant Frank's

floor, he said in a lilting Jamaican accent, "Oh, you a lady friend for Mr. Matheson. He have few lady friends."

What did that mean, exactly? That he had only a few, or that he had many? When Carol got out on the sixteenth floor, the elevator man winked at her.

"Voilà, you have arrived," Frank said as he opened the door to his apartment. He was wearing an apron with a brown cow on the front. "Like my formal evening wear? I ordered this from a French cheese ad."

"Divine," Carol said. "Every man should own one."

The apartment still had a smell of paint and was nearly barren. Frank explained that his old furniture was still in storage. "What I really need," he said, "is a decorator to fix this place up." Through a portal to the left was a spacious living room with a panoramic view of the avenue. Opposite was a beamed-ceiling dining room and a newly renovated kitchen, and down a long hallway was a bedroom.

"It's what I've always wanted," Frank said, leading her into the living room. "A real *city* apartment. I love not having everybody mind your business. You can be anywhere, doing anything, and nobody cares. It's so anonymous."

Carol also liked the anonymity of the city. Then she thought of the elevator man and smiled. "I don't know how anonymous it is for you. Your elevator man seems to know a lot about your life."

Frank laughed lightly. "So Vincent regaled you with tales of my women, did he?"

"How did you know?"

"He tells all my women about all my women," Frank said. "Actually, when a neighbor comes up to borrow coffee, Vincent thinks I'm running a bordello."

"So what's the specialty of the house?" Carol asked.

"Oh, a very complicated meal," he said. "Come to my elegant dining table, dinner's almost ready."

A metal card table with four folding chairs sat in the

middle of the dining room, with the only light provided by the ceiling fixture's bare bulbs. The house
specialty turned out to be steak, baked potato, and
salad, served with store-bought garlic bread, a good
bottle of California cabernet, and a gummy apple pie.
Primitive as the food and the setting were, Carol found
herself enjoying Frank's antics—the flourishes with
which he served the meal, the dumb jokes that made
her laugh.

"So speaking of pets," he said, "who sleeps with
cats?"

"I don't know," Carol said.

"Mrs. Katz."

In chuckling at the inane joke, Carol realized she
must be slightly tipsy on the wine.

"You know Tommy hoots at the way we live," she
said, "in little white boxes. He—"

It was the first time her brother's name had come
up, and Carol instantly regretted having brought him
into the conversation. But he was on her mind, there
was nothing she could do about that—and with the
subject broached, Frank prodded her for progress on
discovering who Paul Miller was.

"I feel funny discussing it with you," she said. "I
know you're Tommy's friend, but . . ."

"Forget it, then," Frank said casually. "But
Tommy's talked with me about it now, so I don't think
he'd mind."

Maybe it was the heavy dinner, the effect of the
wine—she had probably drunk more than half the bottle—but Carol felt completely relaxed with Frank. As
she followed him into the living room, she took pride
in telling how she had discovered that, despite Miller's
claims, the police had never investigated Tommy.

"Is that right?" Frank asked with obvious amazement at her powers of detection. "How do *you* know
that the police don't suspect Tom?"

She had begun to explain prying the information

from Eric Gaines, but suddenly she felt she had gone too far.

Frank, however, was intrigued. "It sounds as if you've spent a lot of time with this cop. Do you think he could be like Miller—using you to get information?"

"I don't think so. He's just a nice guy who knew I was scared."

"I hope you're right. What was this task force thing he took you to see?"

As they sat on the only piece of furniture in the living room, an old leather Chesterfield couch, Carol recounted seeing the wall of maps and photographs at the task force, how horrified she'd been.

"I really admire you for exposing yourself to all that stuff," Frank remarked. "It's courageous."

"Or maybe," Carol said thoughtfully, "I'm a little unbalanced. Maybe I'm as bad as Miller, immersing myself in all this sickness just to be a kind of . . . spy."

"C'mon, it's not remotely the same. I'd say spying to save your brother from a madman is a pretty good cause."

"Thanks," she said, "I needed the reassurance."

Hearing Miller called a madman . . . was that what he was? Carol couldn't be sure any longer who was mad. She leaned back, her eyes closing, and then felt Frank's hand on her arm, sliding up and down.

"Mmmm," he purred seductively.

From the movement of the cushion beneath her, she sensed his body twist as his hand slid languidly over to her neck. She had known he would make a pass, and it was a pleasant feeling. Though it was obviously too soon, she felt she wanted him. His finger delved under the top of her dress, the button opened, and a moment later another. She took in the smell of him again and her skin tensed in goose bumps . . .

. . . until suddenly it seemed very wrong.

In her mind's eye she was seeing the elevator man's

leering wink, hearing his voice . . . *you a lady friend for Mr. Matheson, he have few lady friends.* This wasn't right, she thought. As much as she liked Frank, she had allowed sexual attraction to lead her along, had convinced herself that Frank was a good person when in fact she didn't really know him well enough.

Or was there something else?

Her eyes opened and she sat up, almost toppling him from the couch. She was beyond tipsy, she realized.

"Whoa, what's the matter?"

"I think I ought to be going," Carol said.

"Oh, Carol . . ." There was more than a hint of exasperation in his voice.

She stood up. "Frank, it's not you, I like you . . . but . . . this Miller thing, all the trouble with Tommy . . . I can't keep my feelings straight these days. I'd rather just go home."

There was a moment of tension as he fetched her coat from the closet. He wore a tight frown as he walked her to the elevator. "I've tried my whole repertoire," he said. "Wit, charm, good food, wine. Maybe I should try magic tricks. I used to be pretty good at it as a kid."

Carol mustered her best smile. "Try one more thing for me, will you?"

"For you, anything. What is it?"

"Patience." The elevator door opened. She gave Frank a quick kiss on the cheek and stepped in.

As the elevator closed, Frank was smiling back at her. Under the circumstances, Carol was impressed with how sweet and forgiving his smile was.

18 THE BEETHOVEN SONATA ENDED, the immortal Rubinstein at the keyboard, the announcer said, and the hourly news began. Carol went on drawing, her mind agreeably lost in Dana's conversation with the leader of the Stone-Eating Blokes.

". . . disappearance of a young New Jersey woman one week ago. Neither the police in Morris County or the New Jersey state police—"

The words in the air mingled for a moment with Dana's, then Carol sorted out the voices and the announcer broke through. She laid down her drawing pen and reached over to the radio to turn up the volume.

". . . but at this hour there are no new leads. The woman, twenty-nine-year-old Katharine Middleton, is a dean of counseling at Fairleigh Dickinson University. She was last seen in a university parking lot getting into a car with a man who remains unidentified."

The announcer moved on to a threatened bus strike.

An abduction in a parking lot, one week ago. The week, Carol thought automatically, when Jill had announced her pregnancy and Tommy had received the news so joyfully. Could a man who had just—

No! Carol scolded herself at the direction her mind was taking. She got up from her drawing table. The next couple of hours, if not the whole day, would probably be fruitless, her concentration kaput. She was on her way to the kitchen to make a tuna salad for lunch when the front bell rang.

But the doorman hadn't buzzed her and building security was always rigidly enforced: all visitors must be announced. A neighbor, perhaps?

Carol went to the front door and slipped on the safety chain before opening it a crack.

Eric stood outside.

"Hi," he said through the sliver of an opening.

Instantly Carol felt a jolt of anxiety. If Eric hadn't been announced, it could only mean he had used his police credentials to get past the doorman. And she could imagine only one reason he might present himself behind his professional facade.

"May I come in?" Eric said.

She hadn't made a move to remove the chain, she realized, hadn't spoken—was already erecting her defense. But against what? *He's innocent,* she testified silently to the jury of her conscience, *innocent.*

"Oh . . . sure." She removed the chain and let him in. Leading him to the living room, she said, "You showed the doorman your badge to get up here, didn't you?"

Eric nodded.

"Why?"

"Carol, I'm here because . . . look, can we sit down?"

She wanted to tell him to get out, shout that it was all a mistake and anyone who didn't know that had to be an enemy. But she answered, with quiet formality, "Yes, of course."

He sat on the couch and folded his hands on his lap. Like a priest at a wake, she thought as she sat in the chair opposite him.

"Carol, a woman disappeared last week in—"

"I heard about it on the radio," Carol said tonelessly.

"Ever since you called to ask me about your brother," Eric said, "I've been keeping an eye on all the lists we get from the feds. They're coordinating all state police reports. A new one came in this morning from the state police in New Jersey, and—"

"And Tommy's on it," Carol supplied, and waited—prayed—for Eric to shake his head, dismiss her assumption.

"I figured you ought to be told—that you'd want to know."

She closed her eyes and let her head slump onto her chest. "Oh, God . . . ," she murmured.

"Do you want to hear the details?" Eric asked solemnly.

She raised her head. "Should I?" she asked. The unspoken plea of her mind colored her voice with an imploring tone. *Tell me it isn't necessary, tell me this isn't real.*

"I'm sure you want to help him," Eric said quietly. "Knowing what you're up against is part of putting up the best fight."

"Then tell me."

An hour earlier, Eric said, he had spoken with a Justice Department investigator in Washington who confirmed that the Thomas Warren in their bulletin lived in Saddle River, New Jersey, and was president of his own medical supply company. "I was told that the New Jersey police argued for Tommy to be put on the federal bulletin."

"No wonder," Carol said bitterly, "with a man named Paul Miller going around, mentioning Tommy's name everywhere."

"That could have done it," Eric acknowledged. "I'm sorry, Carol, it's a rotten development." He paused and looked at her, as if weighing how much to say. "This is something that hasn't been given to the papers yet," he went on, "so keep it to yourself. One of the students at the college remembers seeing the missing woman across the parking lot with a blind man— the guy had one of those white canes, and dark glasses. The way this witness tells it, the woman was at a car and seemed to be having some difficulty helping the blind man into the passenger seat. At the time the witness thought it was just the awkwardness of helping a man who couldn't see. But it was night, she was sixty or seventy yards away, and she couldn't be sure. Now she thinks the two people may have been struggling. It fits in, more or less, with the MO we have on Woodsie—excuse me, I mean—"

"It's all right," Carol said. She was almost glad that he would use the callous jargon with her, a sign of trust. "So you think the blindness might have been a disguise, like the crutches."

"Yes."

The image of a man in dark glasses, tapping his cane, formed in Carol's mind. It struck a chord in her somehow, and she lingered over it, trying to bring into focus some vague notion about its significance as a clue.

Eric jarred her out of the reverie. "That's the limit on what we have, though. The witness couldn't give us a description of the car, or recall a thing about the license plate."

"So why," Carol asked, "did this land Tommy on that list?"

Eric shook his head. "They didn't give us any reason, Carol, but it's serious. If he hasn't thought of it already, I think you should tell your brother to get a good lawyer."

Carol stared bleakly at Eric. "You don't think . . . he could be arrested. There's nothing but—"

Eric cut in. "I'm trying to help you, Carol—and help your brother. It's getting to the point that he has to protect himself." He rose and moved toward her chair. She stood up, too. As he reached her, Eric placed his hands on her shoulders. "Carol, you can count on me. I know that anyone who's your flesh and blood is getting a bum rap to be mixed up in this."

Carol saw the tenderness in his gaze and was moved

to respond. Her arms went around his neck, while his slipped down to encircle her waist, and they brought their lips together. But being touched, held—when at the same moment visions of a murderous man in dark glasses still lurked in a corner of her mind—she felt more like a victim than the recipient of real affection. She pulled away.

"Well," Eric said, covering his disappointment, "I'd better get back."

She took him to the door. "Eric, if anything new comes up . . . anything that might help . . ."

"I can't promise," he said, "I've gone too far over the line already." But in the hallway, as he headed for the elevator, he turned back to her. "I'll try, though. I'll do as much as I can."

Tommy's secretary had evidently gone for lunch. The man who answered the phone said that Tommy was also out. "For the rest of the day, I think. He'll be in tomorrow morning."

She nearly telephoned the house in Saddle River, imagining that the New Jersey police might already have taken him into custody. But she didn't want to risk reaching Jill, and if things were that dire, he would have called her.

She went back to her drawing table, but sat there for half an hour without being able to work. The man holding a cane kept tapping his way through her thoughts. . . .

"What on earth is wrong, darlin'?" Margot asked. "You look like Scarlet watching Tara burn."

Carol had given up on work, called the Jenners, and said that she was in need of immediate advice. Margot had said to come straight over. Now Carol followed her to the living room, where Larry stood by the fireplace, a grave, businesslike expression on his face.

Without waiting for the drink Margot was certain to

offer, Carol sat down and told them that her policeman friend had visited her half an hour ago, bringing
bad news. Hearing the details, Larry grew more grave
and Margot shook her head sympathetically.

"It's not good," Carol went on. "The only thing to
do is cut it off before it gets worse. Tommy may need
a lawyer, Larry, and I thought you might be able to
suggest someone."

Larry cleared his throat and looked at Margot. Margot looked at her lap.

Were they already retreating from her? Was this the
price of being linked to someone accused of such horrible crimes? "Look, I only want a recommendation.
You won't be brought into anything—"

"No, no, it's not that," Larry said reassuringly, and
then turned to his wife. "We might as well let her in
on it, Margot."

"Let me in on what?" Carol said.

"As it happens," Larry answered her directly,
"we're having a legal problem of our own just now.
Several of my former colleagues have been indicted
for stock fraud, and they see a way to get clear if they
can leave me holding the bag. But there's no truth to
what they're saying. The lawyer I've retained, a
woman named Myra Cantrell, has been doing a magnificent job. Your problem—I mean Tom's—might be
up her alley."

Carol looked at her friends. "I would never have
guessed you were in this kind of trouble." She turned
and focused solely on Larry. "This lawyer, do you really think she can help? What Tommy's accused of is
so . . ."

"Myra Cantrell has done all kinds of criminal cases.
She's quite the best, Carol, really."

Carol usually thought of criminal lawyers, when she
thought of them at all, as men. But a woman lawyer
for Tommy struck her as ideal. If a woman would de-

fend him, who could believe him guilty of the serial killer's butchery?

"Myra Cantrell sounds just right," Carol said to Larry, and was explaining her reasoning when Adam Jenner and his sister, Kate, banged the front door open.

While Margot shuffled them off to the kitchen, Larry pointed out that the lawyer's ability took priority over her gender. "Being represented by Myra is like having a pit bull in your corner," Larry concluded.

"Will you call her for me?" Carol asked.

Larry picked up a notepad and asked Carol for further details on Tommy's position.

"It looks like I'm going to need a lawyer," Tommy said. "The sooner the better."

A few hours earlier, Tommy reported, Jill had summoned him home from the office. Two detectives from the New Jersey state police had arrived at his house. With his permission they had done a cursory search and questioned him for almost two hours. The time coincided with her phone call to his office, Carol realized. But rather than admit that she had known four hours ago he was in trouble and had tried to reach him—which would mean having to explain her friendship with Eric—she left it unmentioned.

"How's Jill?" Carol asked.

"She's in shock. I called her doctor to ask if it was okay for her to take a tranquilizer—you know, with the baby. He said no."

"And what about you, Tommy?" Carol asked, her tone brimming with concern.

"I can handle it, kiddo. I don't know how the hell I got mixed up in this thing, but there's only one way it can go if I fight back. I asked the company's law firm to recommend a good criminal lawyer, and told them to think about suing this Miller character."

"Let me try to get some recommendations, too,"

Carol said, "maybe from Larry Jenner. He moves in those Wall Street circles, maybe he knows a criminal lawyer." She felt a twinge of guilt at not offering Tommy the solace of knowing she'd found help. But wouldn't he be even more unsettled to know she had felt it necessary to cover his flanks?

Twenty minutes later she was able to call Tommy back to say that Larry had not only recommended an excellent attorney, but had already set up an appointment for the next morning.

19 "MISS CANTRELL WILL SEE YOU NOW," the receptionist said.

Carol stood at her brother's side in the large entrance area of Cantrell, Gassarero & Stein. The law firm's name was mounted in letters of brushed golden metal on the rosewood paneled wall behind the reception desk.

A door to the left of the desk opened, and a striking ash-blond woman stepped out. Myra Cantrell had a bearing simultaneously authoritative and unambiguously feminine. She was very tall—almost too tall, Carol thought, for a woman to be comfortable with, and yet, perhaps precisely because of that, she wasn't intimidating. She wore a beautifully tailored grey suit, but what most held Carol's eye was a pear-shaped piece of jewelry pinned next to the jacket pocket. It seemed modest, but the setting was fine antique silver, and the stones were ruby sapphires. Everything about the lawyer conveyed a sense that she was in charge not only of her life, but also of the world around her.

"Good morning, I'm Myra Cantrell," she said smoothly as she extended a hand toward Tommy. "You're Mr. Warren and this is . . . ?" She turned to Carol.

"My sister," Tommy said. "Carol Warren."

"The children's book author," Myra Cantrell said pleasantly. "Won't you come in."

She preceded them briskly down a long carpeted hallway into a corner office, a large square room with floor-to-ceiling windows on two sides. In the windowed corner was a round Regency mahogany table. On the opposite side, beneath a Warhol print of Mao, was a seating area more like a small living room, with a sofa and chairs upholstered in muted stripes placed on a beige Aubusson rug. On two end tables were framed photographs of Myra Cantrell with the mayor, several U.S. senators, and a group of robed judges— a strong statement of the lawyer's powerful pedigree to go along with her good taste.

"Please sit down," she said. She indicated the sofa for Carol and Tommy and took her place opposite them. "Would you like some coffee?"

Tommy and Carol both declined.

"Well, I'll have some if you don't mind." Myra Cantrell picked up the phone and spoke to a secretary, then turned her attention to Tommy. "Before we talk about your case, I'm wondering why you didn't bring your wife today."

Tommy appeared taken aback. "How did you know I was married?"

"I noticed your wedding ring," the lawyer said matter-of-factly.

Tommy smiled quickly. "Of course. My wife . . . well, the state police put us through some unpleasant questioning. Jill is still pretty rattled. It's happened at a bad time. We've just learned she's pregnant, and we both felt that coming today might be more than she could handle."

"I see," Myra said sympathetically. "How long did the police question you?"

"About an hour and a half. I wasn't sure if I should submit to it, but if I refused . . . I didn't think it would look right."

"It's in your favor that you talked to them. And I think it was wise to let them look at your house and examine your cars."

Carol sat forward. "But don't they need a warrant for that?"

"Technically, yes," Myra replied. "But if Tom had nothing to hide, it's good that he behaved that way." She turned to him. "May I call you Tom?"

"Sure."

"Tom, the police were with you for an hour and a half. Tell me, what points in particular did they dwell on?"

"Mostly where I was the night that woman disappeared and the kind of cars my company owns. Then they asked where I was on other dates, and I said they were welcome to look at my calendar and travel records."

"Did you hand over those records?"

Tommy shook his head. "I started to realize that I ought to have a lawyer."

Myra looked down, as though considering her next question. "As I understand it, you accounted to the police for your time last Thursday."

Tommy sighed. "All I had to do was look at my calendar. I had five appointments starting at eight in the morning, ending with one at four o'clock with a hospital administrator in Cherry Hill, just outside of Philadelphia. We finished at around six, and I got on the turnpike."

"The time we have to be concerned with," Myra said, "is later—around eight o'clock, when a witness says she last saw Kathy Middleton."

"I can cover that. It was rush hour when I got on the turnpike, and I'd been on the road since early in the morning. After an hour of driving I was really exhausted. So I went into one of those rest-stops and had some coffee. I was going to get back on the road, but when I filled up the tank, I still felt whipped. I was afraid to drive, thought I might fall asleep at the wheel."

"How long were you in the restaurant?" the lawyer asked.

"I don't know, maybe half an hour. I read the *Times*, went out to get the gas, then I dozed a little in the car, maybe forty minutes, an hour. Afterwards I got back on the turnpike."

Myra flicked the eraser of her pencil. "So the way it works out," she said, "at eight o'clock you were still taking a nap at the rest-stop. We should be able to check that. Who would have seen you there?"

"I had coffee and bought gas," Tommy said, "so the waitress and the pump attendant might remember me."

"Good. Now, about your calendar and travel records. Don't give them to the police. When the time comes to cooperate, we're going to want some favors in return." She paused. "Let me be clear: I haven't decided yet to take this case. But you should have my views on your wife's not coming today. I can understand it. However, if the police should move beyond questioning—if by some chance there's an attempt to seek an indictment against you—then Jill . . . that is her name . . . ?"

Tommy nodded.

Watching Myra Cantrell, Carol felt the lawyer had no doubt about any such details as names or times or places. She hadn't missed a thing.

Myra continued, "Jill will be crucial to the outcome. I regret the strain on her, but the way you're perceived counts for a lot, Tom. And having her at your side will look very good to a jury, should it come to that."

The lawyer's cold calculations were unnerving enough, but the mention of a jury completely shook Carol's balance. Had things already moved to the point where Tommy was not just fighting off insinuations, but being prepared to go on trial?

The secretary entered with a silver pitcher and three cups and saucers on a tray. The lawyer offered cups to Tommy and Carol and busied herself pouring coffee, plainly tabling discussion of the case until the secretary had left the room.

Tommy spoke as the door closed. "You said you hadn't decided to take my case. Does that mean . . . well, do you doubt me?"

"My reticence doesn't imply that, or anything else. It's simply that I want to know as much as I can before committing myself to a defense."

The phone rang on the table beside her. She held up a finger. "I'm sorry, I've been expecting this one call."

Carol looked at Tommy. He smiled at her and nodded his head up and down, signaling his approval of Myra Cantrell.

"Tell Rodriguez I won't tolerate any more delay," the lawyer was saying into the phone. "If the government has a case, then I'll see him in court." She listened for a moment, then went on. "No way. We're not going to plea-bargain this. You've got twenty-four hours to call me with his answer."

Myra dropped the receiver into its cradle and turned back to Carol and Tommy. "We won't be interrupted again," she said.

Carol had seen other women in influential positions, but none like this, and she read Myra's display of authority on the phone as an encouraging sign. This was the kind of toughness Tommy needed to defeat the allegations against him.

Myra turned to Carol. "Larry Jenner tells me you know a detective working with the state-federal task force on serial killers. Can you tell me how you got to know him?"

Carol was instantly flustered. She hadn't thought that Eric would be brought into this. She launched into a response, anxious to demonstrate there was nothing to hide. But she'd no sooner begun than she noticed Tommy's hurt expression. It must seem to

him, she thought, that she had kept the relationship
hidden because of doubts about his innocence.

When she finished telling Myra how she'd remained
in touch with Eric, the lawyer studied her for a long
moment. She knew, Carol realized, that it was more
than a simple friendship.

But whatever Myra Cantrell had divined, she treated
the issue as only one more factor relating to Tommy.
"Being friends with Detective Gaines is all right. He
may not be so free with information in the future, but
anything you can learn could help. If he does tell you
anything, anything at all, telephone me directly. I'll
give both of you a private line number . . . if I take
the case."

"What will make the difference for you?" Tommy
asked. "What do I have to do?"

"We'll get to that in a minute," the lawyer said, and
walked over to the round table. She picked up the
phone and punched a single button. "Have you found
anything else?" she asked.

While Myra stood at the phone listening, Tommy
glanced at Carol. "I think it's going well," he whispered. "She's very impressive."

Carol nodded. "Tommy, about Eric Gaines . . ."

"Carrie, it's okay, let's talk about it later."

Myra Cantrell had hung up. She walked back across
the room and sat down. "In my practice of law," she
said, "I've spent a great deal of time with people accused of crimes that would turn an ordinary person's
stomach. But the crimes in this case are especially sick-
ening. They violate something fundamental in our
spirit, offend everything in us that's human." While
nothing in the lawyer's tone had significantly changed,
she communicated a new level of seriousness. "Now,"
she said to Tommy, "if you were simply accused of
shooting three people in the head during a holdup,
I wouldn't ask this question—indeed I rarely ask it of
any potential client. But I'm going to ask it of you

now." She looked straight into Tommy's eyes. "Tell me, Tom Warren, are you guilty?"

Carol had guessed what the lawyer would ask. Still, she felt it as a hammer blow to her hold on reality. She saw, too, the shock register in Tommy.

"No," he managed finally, "I'm not. I swear I'm not."

"Fine," the lawyer replied impassively. "Let's move on." She glanced quickly at the paper in front of her. "What I've learned so far is that the police don't have much in the way of evidence. Some vague similarities between your company car and cars that have been identified in the past. And something inconsequential about a license plate. But it does seem that the man Larry Jenner told me about, Paul Miller, has been pushing the police to question you. We don't know yet who he is. One thing we have learned is that he's not associated with federal law enforcement or the state police."

Carol half-raised her hand. "He told me he was working for himself. His daughter was one of the victims."

The lawyer made a note, then asked Tommy, "Are you certain you've never met Miller before—many years ago, perhaps? Is there any reason he might have a vendetta against you?"

Tommy shook his head. "I've racked my brain trying to place the guy. And I'm sure I never saw him until he showed up in my office."

"Can you think of anyone who ever threatened you, said they'd get even with you? Did you fire someone, humiliate anybody in front of a crowd? I assume you've thought about all this, but think again."

While Tommy stared into the middle distance, Myra Cantrell sipped her coffee and watched him. Was this merely a ploy, Carol wondered, a chance for the lawyer to examine Tommy, hunt for some telltale reaction?

"No," Tommy said, "I can't think of anybody."

"Now then . . . there's the matter of doing a line-up in front of the witness to the Fairleigh Dickinson abduction. Have the police explained that to you?"

"Yes," Tommy said. "I told them I was completely willing. Except that I'm concerned about my business. If my name gets in the papers . . ."

"That's been fixed. They wanted to do the lineup later this afternoon. I talked to the chief of detectives this morning and had it switched to nine tonight. There will be fewer people around. I also told them that, if I represented you, you'd be there tonight on the condition that there's no publicity. If we see any reporters, we'll take a walk." The lawyer folded her hands on her lap. "That's where we are. You'll do this lineup and I'll go with you. Bring along your wife if it wouldn't be too rough for her. When we get past this, we'll talk about where we go from here."

"So you're taking the case," Tommy said, brightening.

Yes, the lawyer replied, and without the slightest pause added that she would need a retainer of twenty-five thousand dollars. If a grand jury returned an indictment, there would be an additional retainer of fifty thousand dollars. And should there be a trial, a retainer of a quarter of a million. Carol nearly gasped, at both the mention of a trial again and at the amounts of money.

"A *trial*?" Tommy's voice cracked as he uttered the word.

"I don't believe it's likely," Myra Cantrell said evenly. "But it's standard to let you know all the fees." She stood and opened the office door. "One other thing. There's a forensic psychiatrist I want you to see for a battery of psychological tests. If they show you incapable of certain kinds of crimes, it will be invaluable—enough to convince a jury to acquit you."

Carol suspected that the idea had occurred to Myra

much earlier. An air of improvisation seemed to be part of her technique.

"Whatever you think I should do," Tommy said.

The lawyer smiled, clearly pleased. "I'll set it up."

Tommy thanked the lawyer for agreeing to represent him and assured her the fees wouldn't be a problem. If the worst happened, he said, he could always sell his house.

Myra Cantrell said she doubted such drastic steps would be necessary. She told Tommy to arrive at the state police headquarters tonight no earlier than ten minutes to nine, and to stay in his car until she arrived. She then offered to bring Carol in her own car, and Carol gratefully accepted.

"Very good then. I don't think we have a lot to worry about. Just keep your wits about you, and I'll see you both tonight."

"It's scary as hell," Tommy said in the elevator, "but she makes me feel a lot better."

After a hesitation Carol said, "Tommy, maybe I should've told you about Eric Gaines and me—"

"C'mon, Carrie, it's okay. But you like this detective . . . he's not just some guy you're getting help from, is he?"

How did she describe what she felt? "It's complicated. I do like him a lot, but right now . . . I don't know what the relationship is."

"I hope it turns out okay for you," Tommy said. The elevator doors opened on the first floor. "What do you make of that call," he continued as they walked out to Park Avenue, "the one right after I asked about her taking the case?"

"It sounded like she had somebody in her firm checking what the police have on you," Carol said. "That's all I can figure."

"That's what I think, too. So there must be something on our side." He hugged her. "Thanks for coming. I try to look like I'm doing swell here, but it's more show than go. I can't tell you how much I appreciate all you've done."

"Hey, I love you, you big goof." Carol nearly started to cry. "I'll see you tonight."

He kissed her cheek, then started up toward Fifty-third Street where he had parked his car in a garage.

As Carol walked east across town, her mind went over the scene in the lawyer's office. She was searching for something, a single definitive moment, but not until she had gone several blocks did she realize that what she sought didn't exist.

Myra Cantrell had taken the case. Yet in all her expressions of optimism that things would turn out well, the lawyer—Tommy's first line of defense—had never once said that she believed he was innocent.

20 THE LIGHTS FLASHED ON, harsh floodlamps that made the eight men lined up on stage squint and rear back as if blinded by an oncoming car.

"Face front, please," a voice boomed from a loudspeaker. "Hands straight down at your sides."

The men flattened their hands against their legs, while in a room at the rear, staring through a massive pane of one-way glass, Carol stood watching Tommy, his head tilted against the wall behind him. Her heart surged in her chest. Her brother looked so vulnerable under the lights. He was dressed in a plain sport shirt, and perched on his nose were the black-lens glasses the police had ordered all of the men to wear.

Carol let out a sigh and felt Frank Matheson touch her arm. Having heard from Tommy about the bad turn of events, he had rushed to New Jersey from his last appointment of the day to offer support. A few rows ahead of them sat the witness to the Fairleigh Dickinson abduction, a wispy woman in her mid-fifties, with a plainclothes detective at her side. A housewife taking night extension courses at the university, she had been in the parking lot when the woman who disappeared was helping a man wearing dark glasses into a car.

Carol stared at her. What could the woman see in the darkness then . . . and now?

"Do any of these men look familiar?" The detective's voice filled the dark, claustrophobic room.

The woman rested her elbows on the seat in front of her and leaned forward, peering straight ahead. "I don't want to say anything, not unless I'm . . . I'm very sure. Can they take their glasses off?"

"Glasses off, please," came the detective's deep voice through the loudspeaker.

Carol tensed as Tommy obediently took off the glasses. Each of the other seven men removed the thin wire-frames from their faces.

From the end of the row just behind the detective came another voice. "Captain," Myra Cantrell said firmly, "did this witness ever see the suspect without glasses?"

The detective shot a testy look at the lawyer, then whispered to the woman sitting next to him. She shook her head. The detective picked up the microphone.

"Glasses on again, please," he said in a weary voice.

One for our side, Carol thought.

The witness stood and bent forward. She turned her head far to the left, then to the next man and the next, until her eyes were aimed far to the right at the last man on the stage.

She raised her arm. "I do think," she said, her hand coming up, a finger extended, "that I recognize one of them."

"You're sure?" the detective cautioned her. "You have to stand by what you say. It won't count otherwise."

"Yes, I'm sure now," the woman replied. "I remember how his hair looked, and that's his chin, I'm positive, I'd take an oath on it now." She aimed her finger at the middle of the stage. "It was him, that one."

The "murderer" identified by the witness was, to the obvious dismay of the chief of detectives, a New Jersey state trooper supplied at the last moment to fill out the lineup. Though somewhat similar to Tommy in build, the trooper was stockier, and his features were stronger—a wider face and fuller chin. The police conceded that perhaps a mistake had been made and accordingly lowered Tommy on their list of suspects.

There had been one other piece of good news. Myra Cantrell had learned the results of the forensic examination of Tommy's company car and his sports car. Nothing incriminating had turned up, and the police lab specifically reported that neither car appeared to have been kept especially neat. This, in the lawyer's view, was significant. Too tidy a car, she said, would indicate a guilty man hiding evidence.

"This calls for a celebration," Frank said ebulliently as he followed Carol and Tommy down the steps to the state police headquarters parking lot.

Tommy demurred. "Jill's waiting for me at home," he said. "She needs her own celebration." He turned to Carol. "You and Frank go have dinner on me. After what you've been through with me, you deserve it."

Frank offered to drive Carol into the city, and she walked over to the passenger side of his car.

"No, mine's over there," Frank said, pointing toward the other side of the lot, where another gray Toyota was parked—a four-door version of Tommy's car. Then, in a gesture of collegiate camaraderie, Frank reached out and grabbed the lapels of Tommy's overcoat. "Stay cool, pal. This is going to work out. We're behind you the whole way."

"Thanks," Tommy said. "I really appreciate your coming. Just having you here makes it easier."

He took out his keys and was unlocking his car when Myra Cantrell emerged from the building and walked over to them.

"I need a minute with you and Carol," she said to Tommy.

Frank started to back away. "I'll go wait by—"

"No, you can stay," Tommy protested.

The lawyer seemed on the verge of objecting, but

she went on. "I want to point out that too much optimism at this point is premature. It went very well tonight, but we're not in the clear yet."

"Why not?" Carol asked heatedly. "They said Tommy's not a main suspect."

"That doesn't mean they're going to let up on him." She turned to Tommy. "You may not be under constant surveillance, they don't have enough men for that. But they'll be watching."

Tommy, standing behind the open car door, gripped the metal rim tightly. "I don't get it. Didn't that lineup prove I didn't kidnap anybody?"

Myra Cantrell pulled her fox coat closed. "Let me explain to you how the police think, Tom. Eyewitness testimony is notoriously unreliable. Six witnesses to the same burglary will describe six different burglars. And despite the lab report, the police know a car can be kept free of damaging evidence. More important, they talked to a waitress and a gas station attendant at the turnpike rest-stop. The waitress remembers you, Tom, but she won't say how long you were in there. The pump attendant saw what might have been your car standing in the parking area, but he can't say anyone was sleeping in it. And there's that Birnbaum woman in Connecticut who saw the license plate. Add that to not having alibis for all the disappearances they can document—"

Tommy slapped his hand on the car window. "Holy Jesus," he shouted, "does anyone in the world have alibis for every minute of his life?" He bent over into the car and slammed the driver's seat back, so that it was almost flat. "Look at that, will you? It's one of the reasons I bought these cars for the company. You can recline that seat and go to sleep if you need a few z's on the road. So if the damn pump jockey wanted to see me, he'd have had to come over and look in the damn window. But of course he didn't. He didn't know I was a murderer who needed a fucking alibi!"

Myra put a hand on his shoulder. "Calm down, Tom. Of course nobody expects you to have alibis. I'm only preparing you for how the other side thinks. The police have to build a case against somebody. That's their job." She gently prodded his arm. "Now go on home to your wife and I'll talk with you later in the week."

Tommy kissed Carol and shook Frank's hand, then got into his car and pulled onto the highway. They watched silently as he drove off.

"Let's go," Myra said at last. "It's late."

They started across the lot and had almost reached the lawyer's blue Audi when Carol stopped in her tracks.

A tall figure bundled in a baggy overcoat was headed in her direction, coming down the half-lit steps of the police building. Hatred welled in Carol while in her mind's eye she saw the familiar image: his hand rising to his homburg, the smile, the tip of the hat. But this time was different; the hat stayed on his head and he gave her no smile. Instead he stopped a few feet from her and spoke loudly:

"Carol, I wanted to tell you how much I regret any pain I've caused you. I'm only doing what's necessary."

"You must be Miller," Frank said with a nasty edge. "Leave these people alone." He tugged at Carol's arm. "Ignore him. Keep walking."

But Carol stared at Miller, rigid with fury.

He walked up to her. "I am terribly sorry," he said, reaching to take her hand, "and if there's anything I can do—"

Carol yanked her hand away. "You of all people," she cried out, "you know the pain of your own daughter being a victim. But what you're doing to us is a kind of murder, too. Do you ever think of that? Of what you're doing to our lives."

Myra Cantrell had come up beside them. "Mr. Mil-

ler," she said, "from the little I know about you, I
would guess that you are cognizant of the law. So you
shouldn't doubt that if you persist in harassing my client or his sister, I can and will request that the police
bring charges against you. I suggest you consider my
warning in effect as of this moment."

Miller gave Myra Cantrell a shrewd measuring
glance. Then he tipped his hat and headed away.

Carol felt a burden had been lifted, that Myra's resolve had almost magically succeeded in banishing
this blight from her life.

"I'll get my car," Frank said.

Carol turned to Myra. "Thank you," she said, "and
thank you for taking Tommy's case and treating him
so well tonight."

"He's my client, Carol," Myra responded. "Why
shouldn't I give him the best treatment?"

"I guess I was worried that . . ." Carol broke off, and
then the question that had been lodged in her mind
all day broke from her lips of its own accord. "So you
do believe he's innocent?"

"I've taken the case, period. Innocent people do get
arrested, and some of them are tried and convicted.
But whatever happens, Carol, you must stay away from
Paul Miller. I get the feeling that in his own way, he's
almost as warped as the killer. Many people lose loved
ones, but they don't abandon their lives to vengeance."

"I understand," Carol said.

"Good," Myra said. "Because there's a danger that
anything you say to Miller could get used against Tom,
and we're still in a very tough fight."

Frank pulled up at the corner of Eighty-ninth Street
and Second Avenue. It had rained in the city while
they were gone, and the streets were slick with a fine
sheen, glistening in the glow of the headlights. For a

moment Carol sat in a daze, still trying to absorb all that had happened.

"Would you like to go have a drink?" Frank asked. "Maybe it would help."

Carol was slow to answer. "I'm sorry, I don't think I have the strength to sit in a bar—or for that matter even to talk. Thanks for driving me in."

Frank touched her sleeve as she was reaching to open the door. "Carol, from what Myra said, there's no telling how tough it might get for you and Tommy. So if you need a friend, just someone to lean on, I want you to know I'm here for both of you."

For a split second his concern warmed her, and then she heard another message in his words. "What do you mean, Frank?" she asked sharply. "How tough it *might* get."

Taken aback by her reaction, he fumbled for a response. "I only thought that . . . you can't completely rule out—"

"Rule what out?" Carol asked, bearing down on him.

"Look, Tommy's my friend—the man has done more for me than I'll ever be able to repay. But . . . well, we don't always see people as they really are, do we? Sometimes we only see what we want to see."

"Frank," Carol said with the quiet steadiness of excessive control, "*you* believe in Tommy's innocence, don't you?"

"Of course. But doesn't it make you think just a little with these things the police are saying about the car and the license plate and the alibis?"

"What it makes me think," Carol said, her temper revving, "is that if you care about someone, you get behind them. And if you can doubt Tommy, after what he's done for you, then *that* makes me think you're not a friend. And so you're not the kind of person I'd ever want to lean on. Good night, Frank." She threw the car door open, got out, and marched away, heading toward her building without looking back.

But as she crossed the lobby to the elevator, Frank's words mushroomed and exploded in her mind. If one of her brother's closest friends could defect so easily, then Tommy faced more than an uphill fight. There was still Miller to worry about, and despite Myra Cantrell's skills, she had twice refused to affirm his innocence. The lawyer's battle, Carol thought, was not for Tommy so much as it was for herself . . . for her desire to win. He was a client, nothing more. Even Jill had wavered.

So there was no one who believed wholeheartedly in Tommy's innocence. No one—except herself.

IN THE
DEEP
WOODS

The birds were suddenly silent.

That had never happened before . . . or had it?

Running through memories of other times, he leaned back, pulling the knife free as he did, and he gazed up at the lacing of branches above him. Seeing the boughs of yellow leaves flicking across the sunlight as they rustled in the breeze, he was reminded of camera shutters, each intermittent stab of light like a flash bulb going off. Hey now, wouldn't that be something—if there could ever be pictures of him at a moment like this.

But what had made the birds stop twittering? Had they all flown away? Terrified perhaps? Yet that was no judgment against him, he realized, no more than the fleeing of smaller jungle creatures from the place where the lion dragged down the gazelle. It was all part of nature's design. The strong affirmed their place in the order by preying on the weaker. Killing had to be part of the plan. That was why it had to be done here in a corner of wilderness. Here, his urge was understood. In other parts of the world he always felt secretly out of place, always had to hide this most basic part of his nature. But deep within the forest it was all right to kill.

Better than all right: it was expected.

Beneath his straddled legs there was a tiny movement, a twitch. He looked down again into her eyes. The sparkle was gone, clouded over, and the lids were half-closed, but she was still conscious, trying somehow to send a silent message. To him . . . or to God, he thought. Or weren't they both the same at a moment like this?

He smiled at her and simply shook his head. Then he held the blade in front of her eyes again before slowly moving it

*down, touching just the pointed tip of it to the cleft between
her breasts, then at another place on her stomach, then lower.
By now of course she knew the knife would go in somewhere,
and weakened as she was by the loss of blood, she still whim-
pered and gave a wan flinch at each pricking touch.*

*At last he pushed down, penetrating her body again. Though
muted by the cloth across her mouth, this moan of pain was
still louder than the others.*

*This time he had chosen to go for something vital. She
wouldn't live more than another few minutes, he guessed. He
rose to get the other things he needed.*

*Then, as he was leaning over the array on the oilskin, he
was struck by a strange sensation, an odd unsettling confusion
he had never experienced before. A feeling of being slightly lost,
of not being sure . . . whether to go on.*

*He glanced over his shoulder at the figure on the ground,
sun and shadow playing over ivory skin and the slick reflecting
stripes of wet blood. And it occurred to him that if he stopped
now, maybe he could stop forever. Maybe it was time. Could
he go on and on without someday pushing beyond an acceptable
limit of risk? Obviously he was already in some danger. If he
walked away this minute, made this one the last—indeed, left
it unfinished as proof of control over his will—then the danger
would be over.*

*So what would be left of his life? He would exist as an ordi-
nary man, like any other. Doing his job. Paying his bills. Taking care of petty affairs. Day after day passing . . . while all
the while, to the day of his own death, he would be denying
the part of him that the animals, at least, could easily understand.*

*The confusion passed, a moment of crazy doubt that he
vowed never to tolerate again. For him the risks would always
be manageable. He picked up the hatchet and walked back to
the girl.*

*As he raised his arm over her neck, he was aware of a couple
of birds chirping again in the tree just overhead.*

21 "FORGIVE THE MESS, but we're just putting in some new sliders for the sun porch—hoping to beat winter." The young woman led Carol down three steps into a sunken living room, setting the tray she was carrying on a coffee table consisting of a slab of amber glass supported by low brass legs.

Carol stood back for a moment, surveying the wall of heavy plastic sheeting that blocked the otherwise empty doorframes. Beyond lay a view of Long Island Sound, reduced to a murky blur by the plastic. Considering the cold air blowing in around the edges, it would have made more sense to have coffee in the kitchen, but from the moment Carol appeared at the door of the house, there had been a nervous effort to extend full hospitality. As the mother of three young children, Lisa Birnbaum had recognized Carol's name as soon as she heard it on the phone, and she had offered no resistance to Carol's unexplained request to come to Connecticut and talk to her personally.

"The youngest one isn't reading yet," she'd said during the call, "but the twins have all the Dana books. I'd be absolutely delighted to meet you." Of course, Lisa Birnbaum had also asked at least four times what they had to talk about, but Carol had dodged the questions, saying only it was a personal matter.

"Good Lord," the other woman had said at last, "I hope you're not going to tell me you're Dave's mistress." There was a perky brightness to her tone that indicated she wasn't really worried.

Carol had laughed. "No. It's nothing that will make you unhappy."

Now Lisa Birnbaum was kneeling behind the glass-topped table, unloading a china coffeepot, cups, saucers, napkins, spoons, and a plate of petits fours from the tray. Carol took a seat on the blue velour sectional sofa.

"This is such a wonderful mystery," said Lisa Birnbaum, "having you call like this. I told a lot of my friends about it. Most of them have kids, so they know who you are."

Carol smiled. But now that she was here, she felt as constrained as she'd been on the phone. She had believed then that if she admitted what she wanted, Lisa Birnbaum might prefer not to become further involved. So Carol had postponed it, and she still didn't know quite how to begin.

"Milk and sugar?" asked Lisa. She was in her early thirties, pretty except for a slightly coarse complexion left over from adolescent acne. Her light brown hair was held back with a tortoiseshell clip, and she was wearing pale stone-washed jeans with a tailored blouse of burgundy silk.

"Just milk," Carol answered.

Lisa Birnbaum added milk, handed the cup and saucer across the table, and told Carol to help herself to the pastry. "Okay, Carol, c'mon: the suspense is killing me."

Carol sought one more postponement in a sip of coffee. Then she put the cup down.

"Mrs. Birnbaum—Lisa—please forgive me for imposing on you this way, but right now you're the person who can help me most with a very serious problem."

Lisa Birnbaum raised her eyebrows in surprise. She had remained on the far side of the low table, and now she informally settled on the floor with her feet tucked under her.

"I wanted to see you," Carol went on, "because something you told the police is the most important piece of evidence in a situation . . . in causing my brother to come under suspicion for something he didn't do."

Lisa Birnbaum's face lost its look of perky expectancy and turned to a somber mask. Seeing the transformation, Carol felt suddenly ashamed, as though she had invaded the woman's home under false pretenses.

"He's absolutely innocent," Carol rushed on, "he's just one of twenty or thirty suspects caught up in this nightmare, but he's in trouble now, and I thought if I could talk to you, learn more about what you saw, there was a chance something would turn up that rules him out."

With pain-stricken eyes Lisa Birnbaum went on staring at Carol for a moment, then looked away through the portal of her living room, as if checking her house to make sure everything was secure.

"Please," Carol said, a fluttery quality entering her voice. "I know how unpleasant it must be for you to be involved in something like this. But I can't go anywhere else for this information."

Slowly, Lisa Birnbaum turned to face her again. "They've been here seven or eight times already. Police and . . . men from some group, a task force. They came one night when I was giving Emmy a bath—my daughter—and Dave wasn't here, so I couldn't leave her. Can you imagine—they stood at the bathroom door the whole time and asked their questions. And they kept telling me how important it was, they always tell me that, because of what this man has done, the terrible things." She bit her lip and Carol leaned forward, ready to reach out, but Lisa Birnbaum shied back. "In front of my little girl, you see . . . they talked

about it right in front of her. That's why I just
wish . . ." Her voice trailed off.

"It is awful," Carol said. "You didn't ask to get
pulled in, and it's . . . such an ugly thing. But it's the
same for me. And for Tommy, my brother. He didn't
ask for this. It just happened, because . . . well, it's
partly that license plate you saw."

Lisa Birnbaum was wringing her hands, her head
bowed over them. Abruptly she looked up, and now,
mixed with her discomfort, there was a wariness in her
eyes. "How did you find me?" she asked flatly.

The question was inevitable. Last night, after the
lineup, Carol had realized that only one witness figured prominently in the case against Tommy. Myra
had mentioned a woman from Connecticut named
Birnbaum, and Paul Miller had described a witness
from Rowayton who had recalled part of a license
plate. Putting the two together, Carol had obtained
the phone number from Connecticut information.

"You were mentioned by a private investigator,"
Carol said, "and also by a lawyer who's talked with the
police. You're entitled to privacy and I've unfairly invaded it, but don't you see how badly I need your
help?"

After a moment Lisa Birnbaum's face softened into
a look of compassion. "Ask me whatever you want to
know."

"Thank you," Carol said.

They exchanged brief smiles. A bond had been
formed, a recognition of their shared plight as victims.

Unaccustomed to the role of interrogator, Carol felt
awkward. "The thing I keep wondering is how you
happened to see this license plate. When I was told
there was a witness, it was also mentioned that you'd
only gotten an impression of the registration number."

Lisa nodded, apparently agreeing. "It's funny the
way memory works, isn't it? I happened to see the car,

but I didn't know I was going to have to remember anything, that it would turn out to be important. It was only later, when the police asked me to look back and try to remember, that certain things stuck in my mind."

Carol took one of the petits fours. Though not hungry, she was anxious to keep the mood relaxed. Crazy as it might be, she actually feared that Lisa Birnbaum's attitude would change if her hospitality was snubbed.

"Maybe you could start by telling me where and how you saw the car?"

"Sure." Lisa also took one of the small cakes. "These are good, aren't they?"

"Delicious." Carol waited for her answer.

Lisa took a bite, sipped her coffee. "My niece, Connie, had her appendix out a couple of months ago, up in the hospital at Stamford. I went over one evening to spend some time with her, and I stayed until visiting hours were over—that's how I was able to tell the police the time, it had to be only a little after nine o'clock when I left. Walking across the parking lot to my car, I saw a nurse standing and talking to a nice-looking young man by another car, several spaces away from mine. Just as I came along, the man opened the passenger door and the nurse got in—it looked like he was offering her a ride somewhere. That's all there was to it. They drove off, so did I. The only reason I remembered it later was that the nurse was one of the people who'd been taking care of Connie. So when I read in the paper a month later that she'd disappeared, it came back to me. I called the police in Stamford, and they sent a couple of detectives out here to talk to me."

"And you described the man and the car for them." Lisa nodded.

"How did you describe the man?"

Lisa pondered. "Nice-looking, like I said—pretty

slim and well built, on the tall side, and he seemed to have brown hair."

"Seemed?" Carol asked.

"Well, it was nighttime. So I really couldn't be sure of the color."

"Lisa, from what you've told me, it doesn't sound like you could have had a very good look at the license plate either. The other car was parked several spaces away and—"

"No, I saw the license number very well. Because when I drove out of the lot, the other car was right ahead of me."

"Okay. But what about remembering it for a month or two?"

"Well, I didn't remember all of it."

Before Carol could pursue the point further, there was a series of percussive noises from the kitchen—cupboards being slammed, glasses clinking, a clatter of footsteps.

"My twins," Lisa said, playfully rolling her eyes, "home from school. Excuse me." She bounded up from beside the table and left the room. The noise from the kitchen subsided and Lisa returned in a minute.

"They're a sideshow," she said. She seated herself again, this time on the other end of the sectional from Carol. "I'd like you to meet them . . . but maybe not while this is in the air."

Carol nodded understandingly. "You were saying you didn't remember all of the registration number."

"No."

"But you told the police that you had an impression of it."

"Right. Three numbers, followed by three letters."

Driving up to Rowayton, Carol had been acutely conscious of all the license plates she had seen—many from New York and Connecticut, some from New Jersey, a few from Pennsylvania and other states. The combination of three letters and three numbers was much too common to be incriminating. So it came down to the one specific detail Lisa Birnbaum had been willing to give the police.

"But you were sure about two of the numbers," Carol said.

"Uh-huh. The two eights."

Carol shook her head, perplexed. "I don't see how that's possible, Lisa—I mean, to be certain of anything. It was dark that night, and even if the car was in front of you for a while, by the time you had to think about it, a month had passed."

"The twins," Lisa Birnbaum said. "I remembered because of the twins."

Carol stared at her dumbly.

"Well, they're nine now—it was their birthday just last week. But they were eight at the time this happened. And when I saw the license plate . . . well, it just stayed with me for that reason. Twin eights." She smiled sheepishly.

Carol took a deep breath. A wave of despair swept through her. It was the sort of detail, she imagined, that could sway the minds of policemen—or if it came to that, a jury. Because of the coincidence of her children's age, a mother would remember two numbers on a license plate. Carol pushed her cup away.

"You've been very patient and cooperative, Lisa. I appreciate it."

"I'm sorry if it didn't help, Carol."

Carol stood and Lisa Birnbaum rose to escort her out. The twin eights hovered in her mind, an image like two sentries guarding the way to the truth, or like handcuffs—

Suddenly another side of the coincidence struck her, and she turned back quickly. "Lisa, you said it's because of your twins that you remembered."

"Yes . . ."

"But suppose because of the twins your mind

played a different kind of trick. Isn't it possible that you took two images that were similar, but not identical, and then twinned them?"

"Sorry, Carol, I don't follow."

"Well, say what was really on the license plate was a B and an eight. They'd look pretty similar, wouldn't they? Or in a quick look, even a three might look like an eight. Or an S. Do you see? Maybe you just took one eight and paired it in your mind . . . because of the twins."

As she gazed back at Carol, Lisa Birnbaum's mouth subsided into a thoughtful frown. "You know, I guess it's possible," she said after a few moments. "For a whole year those same two numbers were in my head all the time. So . . . maybe that's how it worked."

"And you'll tell the police if they ask? You'll tell them you're not sure anymore?"

"Of course I will. That's the truth."

Impulsively, Carol hugged Lisa Birnbaum. "That's all I needed, Lisa. That should do it for Tommy."

22 CAROL RETURNED LATE TO THE CITY. Giving autographs to the Birnbaum twins had led to a plea from Lisa to stay for dinner and meet her husband, an executive with a New York manufacturer of costume jewelry. On impulse Carol had accepted the invitation, feeling a need to remind herself what it might be like if a day came when she was no longer alone—when she had a husband and children and a house that needed its windows replaced.

When she left, Carol knew—despite the heartfelt pledges on both sides to keep in touch—that she was unlikely ever to see the Birnbaums again. But she brought home more than an expectation that Tommy would soon be cleared; she returned with a conviction that her world would be normal again.

Opening the door of her apartment, she saw a light burning in the entrance hall. Had she turned it on this morning, perhaps by accident on her way out? She took a cautious step inside. Along the hallway she could see a soft glow emanating from another light in the bedroom.

"Hello . . . ?" she called tentatively.

For a few seconds there was no answer, then Carol heard noises from behind the closed door of the bathroom. She took a single step backward, then the door swung open and a figure in billowing white emerged and rushed toward her. It took a second before she realized it was her sister-in-law wearing a nightgown.

"Jill! How long have you been here?"

"Only an hour, I . . . didn't know when you'd be back." Wet from a shower, Jill's hair was splayed wildly around her head. "Maybe I shouldn't have come," she said in a plaintive voice. "But I needed a place for tonight."

It sounded as if she were begging permission. Yet Carol had long ago given a key to Tommy and made it clear that he or Jill could use the apartment if they found themselves in the city and couldn't reach her. A terrible intuition began to take shape, but before Carol could give it words, Jill went on.

"I've left him. Tomorrow I'm going up to Vermont to stay with my folks."

Carol sighed. "Of course you can spend the night here." She moved toward Jill, reaching out, hoping that a show of sympathy would unite them enough so that she could reason with her. But Jill pulled away.

Still hoping to talk, Carol went into the living room and switched on a lamp. Waiting for Jill to take the cue, she puttered idly, stripping petals from a bunch of wilted yellow tulips in a vase on the end table.

Jill followed her into the room. "You hate me for it, I suppose."

"No, none us could go through this without having some trouble. There've been times when even I . . . when I gave in just enough to wonder if anything is impossible, gave in for just a second. I think it would be sad, though, if we let our doubts rule us for any longer than that."

There was a silence. Jill moved up close behind Carol. "You know what I think, Carol?" She came still closer, and when she spoke next, standing right at Carol's shoulder, there was a force to her words no less brutal than if she had swung a club. "I think Tommy did everything they say."

Carol whirled on her sister-in-law. "My God, how can you . . . ?"

"Because suddenly it makes everything so clear," Jill replied quietly. She began to pace, not back and forth but weaving an irregular pattern across the open floor, through all the spaces between the furniture. "Like the baby. He never wanted one, did you know that? For years I couldn't wait to start a family, but he kept putting me off."

"He's devoted himself to the business," Carol came back quickly. "You're both young enough that it was possible to wait a few years. He might have been playing it down for your sake, too, keeping the pressure off. You had some fertility problems, didn't you?"

"Yes, there were problems. But we looked into all that with a doctor, and he helped us . . . told us things to do, you know. But for a long time Tommy wouldn't do any of it. My fertile days would come, and he just wouldn't be around."

"Jill, how can you make that a reason for such terrible doubts? It's hard to make love on a schedule."

"Sure, I'll accept that. But suddenly Tommy changed—he was there just when the doctor ordered. And you know when that was, Carol, when he got real hot on this baby idea? Two or three months ago, that's all. Just when he might have found out that he was a suspect!" Jill spun around and went to the window, stared out at the city.

Carol targeted a chilling gaze at her sister-in-law. "For God's sake, Jill," she said, "can you really believe Tommy suddenly wanted a baby because he thought it would make him look more innocent? He was ready, that's all. Ready for something you both want!"

Jill kept facing the window as if shouting into the night. "Carol, he told me: that lawyer, the woman who's representing him—she could see right away how it might help, told him it might look good to a jury."

"Oh, Jill . . ." Pity came at last as Carol saw how any joy in the baby had been subverted—aborted—by the demon of Jill's own suspicion. "Do you think if Tommy were guilty he would have told you Myra said that? The truth is, he was a little shocked when he heard that—we both were. Naturally he doesn't like the idea of using you that way—doesn't like to think it might ever come to that. But the idea didn't come from him. He's scared, too, don't you see? Just the way you are, the way I was."

Carol's use of the past tense seemed to hit the air like a sonic boom. Jill turned to her again. "So if you were scared, how did things change for you?"

"I found out today that some of the information responsible for putting Tommy on that suspect list—maybe the most important detail—isn't reliable."

Jill cocked her head, obviously eager to hear more.

Quickly Carol reported on today's trip to Connecticut, Lisa Birnbaum's admission that her memory of the license plate could be faulty. "Without that number, Jill—those two eights—there's really no evidence against Tommy, nothing with any substance."

But Jill shook her head, and a tight smile touched her lips. "It isn't going to go away now, Carol, not that easily. Maybe you've given that woman second thoughts, but you can't be sure she was wrong."

"Good God, Jill, don't you think your husband deserves the benefit of the—"

"I'm not the only one," Jill rushed on. "There are plenty of others who've had their eyes opened. Tommy's own secretary quit two days ago, and another girl in the office."

Carol winced, and her mouth fell open in a silent gasp.

Jill caught the signs of surprise. "So you didn't know, huh? Tommy didn't tell you that there are women who are so scared to be near him that they can't work anymore." She moved up on Carol. "But

that's not all. He was called into the bank yesterday—
the one in Flemington where the business has a bridge
loan for three hundred thousand dollars—and they
told him they wanted it repaid right away. Tommy was
able to buy some time, but only by promising to step
down from the company until he's proven innocent.
He had to put Frank in charge. You see, Carol, I'm
not alone."

"It's a witch-hunt, that's all!" Carol started to pace.
Then, to keep herself collected, she forced herself
down onto the sofa. "There's nothing against him, Jill.
People are just easily frightened, banks don't want to
take a chance." Her voice broke. Fighting harder to
hold herself together, she pushed the words out.
"Damn it, this is what's so awful. The system tells us
over and over we're innocent until proven guilty—but
every damn time it works the other way. Just get
touched by the edge of a shadow, and all anyone can
see is the dark spot."

Jill came over to the sofa. Very quietly she said,
"There's something else, Carol. Something I
found . . ."

Carol turned to her sister-in-law. "Found?" she echoed.

Jill hesitated, then walked out of the room. Carol
was left wondering if she had simply quit talking.

But in half a minute she returned, a strip of colorless
cloth dangling from her hand as she came back toward
the sofa. "A couple of weeks ago," she said, "I was fixing up a space in the attic to use for a study, and I went
looking for some leftover paint to touch up an old
bookshelf. Down in the basement, in the paint closet,
this turned up."

Carol pulled the piece of cloth from Jill's grasp. It
was a strip of coarse unbleached linen, two or three
inches wide and perhaps a couple of feet long, rumpled a little at each end. An innocuous thing. For the
first time it occurred to Carol that maybe the strain

of dealing with Tommy's problem had crippled Jill's ability to see anything clearly.

"There's nothing odd about keeping bits of cloth in a paint closet. When I was a kid, we always—"

"Carol, look at it!" Jill grabbed it back. "This isn't just some torn-up old rag for cleaning brushes. It's been carefully cut. And it wasn't the only one in the closet. There were eight or nine others just like it, some with creases in them. At first I didn't make anything more of it. But once I started thinking, I saw another side."

"What did you make of it then?" Carol said evenly.

Jill held the cloth up in front of Carol's eyes. "You see the way it's wrinkled at the ends? That comes from their being tied in a knot." Jill took the two ends, tied them together, and formed a loop. "This is too short, but if you linked a couple together it would be twice as big."

"And . . . ?"

"Carol, the police said the killer does something to put his victims off guard, make them think he needs help."

Carol nodded. "They think he uses crutches sometimes."

"And what about *this?*" Jill slipped the circle of cloth over her head, then hooked her arm through it. The loop was too small, too awkward to work, but Carol got the idea. Two lengths of the cloth tied together would form a sling.

"Did you ask Tommy about it?" Carol said.

Jill looked at her askance. "How could I? I didn't even want him to know I'd found it."

"So he doesn't get a chance to explain. No defense." Carol pulled herself to her feet. "You know what else you could make with those strips, Jill? A noose for a lynch mob. Because that's what's happening to Tommy now. He's being lynched. By you, by those women at work, the bank. He doesn't have a chance. Not if you're going to find some rags in a paint closet and make them the reason to leave him when he needs you most."

"Carol, you can't just close your eyes to the—"

Carol kept heading out of the room. "That's exactly what I have to do," she said wearily. "Close my eyes, go to sleep, and make sure I wake up with a clear head. Because if there's anything I can see right now, it's that my brother's going to need me at my best. Use the sofa bed, Jill. You know how to set it up."

She stalked out and went into her bedroom.

Slumped onto the bed, Carol brooded about losing her temper with Jill. But she felt worse about the problems Tommy was having. She grabbed up the phone, hoping to provide some relief for him.

"Is Jill with you?" Tommy asked as soon as they'd exchanged hellos.

"Yes."

"I wish she could understand."

"Give her time. Being away may be just what she needs."

"The funny thing is that I can't blame her—with her husband accused of . . . of this kind of thing, and the baby coming. I think it's been even harder on her than on me."

"It may blow over soon," Carol said. "I have some good news for you." She launched into a report of her success with Lisa Birnbaum.

When she had finished, Tommy was pleased but wary. "Carrie, it's a fantastic thing you've done, but be careful with this stuff, will you? Let Myra handle it. I don't want you getting in trouble."

"If I can't get in trouble for you," she asked, "who should I get in trouble for?"

"You told Jill what you found out, I hope."

"I told her," Carol said, sorry that she couldn't add that it made some difference.

Tommy read her inflection. "Doesn't she realize it helps put me in the clear?"

Carol paused, oddly restrained by the notion that she was violating Jill's confidence. But then she explained about Jill's discovery of the linen strips and the significance she attached to it.

It was a long time before Tommy spoke again. "I get it," he said quietly. "She thinks it fits into the police theory about the killer's disguises. Is that why you're really calling—to tell me this, Carrie? Because you need an explanation, too?"

"No!" she cried. "I just want you to know what you're up against."

He went on in a level voice. "I had an old piece of canvas. I cut it up to make—"

"Tommy, don't. Please."

He stopped. "I'm sorry, Sis," he said softly. "But it's getting to me. My secretary quit." He let out a despairing little laugh. "Even the women who haven't quit leave early every night. They don't want to get caught in the parking lot after dark. Do you suppose Jill might wait to see me? I'll be at your place around noon tomorrow . . . you know, I have that appointment Myra arranged." He was going to see the forensic psychiatrist at two o'clock and Carol was going with him.

"I don't think Jill will stay, Tommy."

He said nothing, and a lump rose in Carol's throat.

"It's bad now," she said, desperate to comfort him, "but it'll come out okay in the end."

"Promise?" he asked, the question of a little boy spoken with the weariness of an adult.

"Cross my heart," she said.

She made a point of rising early to make breakfast for Jill. By the light of day, over cups of coffee, Carol felt there was a chance of prevailing on her sister-in-law to give Tommy another chance.

But on the way to the kitchen she saw that the sofa

bed was empty, and she noticed then that Jill's big valise was gone.

The crippling of Tommy's marriage left Carol feeling angry—more at Miller than at Jill—and though she
tried to retreat into her work, every attempt failed.
Several times she went to the drawing table, looked
over unfinished sketches or line drawings that needed
to be colored, then got up to wander around again.

On her third or fourth restless tour of the apartment, she noticed the knotted loop of linen Jill had
left lying on the coffee table. She picked it up, turned
it in her hand a moment, then slipped it over her neck.

Yes, a couple of them strung together would be long
enough for a sling. And the police knew already that
the killer disarmed women by disguising himself as
disabled. A man with his arm in a sling might be able
to plead for help as believably as a man on crutches.

She flung the loop of cloth down again and returned
to the drawing table.

And then she became aware of some half-formed
thought shimmering in the recesses of her mind like
a bright object submerged in murky water. Something
about the sling—

No, not the sling. But about this theory of disguises—the killer making himself appear helpless and
harmless. As in that recent case, when a witness had
seen a woman being abducted by someone who appeared to be blind.

In some undefined way the image of the killer feigning blindness struck Carol as a kind of breakthrough.
In her mind she conjured a man in dark glasses, black
lenses. If she could only strip those glasses from the
face in her vision, she would truly see the face of the
guilty man.

And then suddenly it came to her. But it wasn't the
glasses that had given him away, she realized.

It was the cane. The blind man's white cane.

23 "IT ALL FITS. The cane, the talent for mime . . ."

Carol was walking up Second Avenue with Margot.

"What about the car?" Margot asked.

"Frank drives a company car," Carol said, "the same kind Tommy has. Maybe he even used Tommy's car. That would account for the license plate."

Margot took a bite from the bagel she was holding. "Darlin', do you remember what you told me, the first time you went out with Frank? How he was so interested in this Miller character?"

Carol shook her head in amazement. "Even *then* I thought it was strange, that's why I mentioned it to you. And that night he cooked dinner for me, that was another strange one. Lots of small talk about the elevator man, needing a decorator to fix up the apartment, but he was soft-soaping me. He turned the conversation around to Miller again, and he grilled me about Eric, wanted to know everything I knew."

They waited at the corner of Eighty-ninth Street for the light to change.

"I keep seeing him at Tommy's party, too," Carol said. "Doing his Chaplin routine with a little bowler hat and a white cane—a blind man's cane cut off at the bottom. Then at the lineup, that number about what a pal he is. Maybe he went with us that night to check out the witness, see what she knew."

"What a pal," Margot said. "He must have been

praying Tommy would get picked." The light changed, and they started across. "Who could frame you better than a friend?" Margot went on. "Frank must know Tommy's schedule, he can call the office and find out where Tommy is, when he'll be back."

As they reached the other side of the street, Carol saw Tommy's car backing into a space across from the canopy of her building. She ran over as he got out.

"Did Jill leave?" he asked before she could say a word.

"I couldn't stop her, Tommy."

Tommy's expression clouded.

Margot came up beside them. "Did you tell him?"

"Tell me what?" Tommy said.

"I think you're being framed," Carol said. "And I think I know how."

"It's absurd," Tommy said, perched on the edge of the couch, "you're reaching too hard. I've known Frank for six years. If he's a murderer, then I'm the man in the moon."

"Funny," Carol replied, "that's almost what he said about you. Sang your praises up and down. Except that he changed his tune as soon they were really after you."

Tommy let out a dry laugh. "You two are incredible. Frank does a Charlie Chaplin routine and on that you're ready to convict him."

"Jesus," Carol cried impatiently, "the cane! The witness saw a blind man. Frank's got the cane—and he's a brilliant mime."

Tommy just shook his head.

Carol went on. "How can you defend him? Look at what he's doing to you after the way you helped him. You took a sales manager and boosted him up to—"

Tommy had stood. "Is that what Frank told you, that he was a sales manager at Bio-tech?"

"Yes," Carol said.

"He was a *salesman,*" Tommy said slowly, pacing behind the couch. "I don't get it with Frank sometimes."

"What are you talking about?" Carol asked.

"When he came to work for me at Bio-tech he'd goosed up his resume a little. I called for a reference and it turned out he'd added ten grand to his salary and inflated his title." Tommy let out a faint whistle. "Later I found out he made up some honorary award in college."

Carol was dumbfounded. "How could you hire a man who lied on his resume? How could you trust somebody—"

"Hold on, Carol. I hired him because he's a great salesman and a terrific manager. And it's a big step from lying on a resume to killing thirty or forty women. Okay, so maybe Frank gilded the lily a bit. Half of America fixes parking tickets and cheats on their income tax."

Margot had been sitting quietly on the arm of the club chair. She leaned forward now. "Tommy, did Frank ever take your company car on a sales call?"

Tommy put his hand to his face and stroked it thoughtfully. "A couple of times. I use my own car a lot, so sometimes my company car's free."

"You see," Margot said triumphantly. Rising from her chair, she strode across the room. "I wonder, if we could get into his apartment, we might find something there."

"What if I called Frank?" Carol said. "If I could get him talking, maybe he'd say one thing, just a slip of the tongue."

"Stop!" Tommy exclaimed. "Both of you. What do you think this is, a Nancy Drew mystery? Two girls going after a killer? I don't believe Frank is guilty of anything. But if he were, the last thing you should do is play detective. We'll tell Myra and she'll get the cops to investigate."

Margot was pacing, ignoring Tommy. "You said he

needed a decorator, Carol. What if I called him and pretended—"

Tommy spun on her. "Margot, cut it out! You're scaring the hell out of me!" His outburst had the effect of yanking them back to reality. For a moment everyone was silent. Then Tommy said, "There's one other thing to consider. Suppose you're right about Frank. If you did find some piece of evidence, we probably couldn't use it anyway."

"Why not?" Margot asked.

"Remember that guy accused of killing his wife with a drug overdose? The woman's daughter asked some lawyer friend to search the family mansion—up in Rhode Island, wasn't it? And when the guy went on trial, the jury didn't believe the evidence. Because it was found by a friend. Better if Myra can pressure the police to do it."

"Oh, sure," Margot said derisively. "You think the cops'll go right in and find the evidence? They'll question Frank first . . . and that'll give him a chance to destroy it."

"Myra's a lawyer," Tommy replied forcefully. "She does this every day. Let her make the choice."

"He's right, Margot," Carol said.

Tommy was already at the phone. He asked for Myra Cantrell, then gave his name to the secretary and hung up.

"Myra's in court all day," he said, "I'll try her later. In the meantime, you two forget any harebrained schemes. I don't accept this stuff about Frank, but if by any chance you've hit on something, you could get yourselves killed." He went to the foyer and took his coat from the closet. In a milder tone he added, "I appreciate what you're trying to do, but let Myra handle it. Okay?"

"Whatever you want," Margot said, defeated.

"Thank you," Tommy said. He put his coat on. "Let's go, Carol. I don't want to be late."

*   *   *

Herbert Gray's office was on the ground floor of a brownstone on West Seventy-first Street off Central Park West. The psychiatrist met them himself at the steel-gated door. Carol had expected an elderly man, assuming that anyone in a field as arcane as forensic psychiatry had spent years in apprenticeship. But Herbert Gray was in his mid-thirties, with regular features and reddish hair styled in feathery layers. He could have been one of those young-married types in a coffee commercial.

Carol had thought she would simply leave Tommy when they arrived, but Gray invited her to join them. They went into a large airy office with dark paneling and an old partner's desk in the center of the room. Circling the desk, the psychiatrist sat down. Carol took a chair next to Tommy on the other side and watched Gray toy with a gold pen, twirling it between his fingers as if he were a magician palming a coin.

"Well, here we are. Any questions?"

Tommy said, "You know what this is about."

"Certainly. Myra told me."

Tommy shifted uncomfortably in his chair. "Then you know a lot's riding on this. Maybe my whole life."

"Perhaps that's an exaggeration," Herbert Gray said in a friendly way.

Carol was leery of asking questions, certain that her behavior would be judged, factored into any appraisal of Tommy. Yet shouldn't the psychiatrist understand that some anxiety was reasonable? "I was wondering," she said, "if you could tell us how this works, what you can really learn about a person."

"I'd be glad to," Gray said. "The first thing to keep in mind is there's no pass or fail. This isn't an exam, but a series of exercises. One, the real granddaddy, is the Rorschach—the inkblots I'm sure you've seen before. There's also a newer exercise called the Thematic Apperception Test, or TAT as it's known in the

trade. It involves looking at some pictures to see what
a person thinks about them. Then we play some games
with numbers, put some puzzles together. And that's
it."

Tommy glanced at Carol, then at the doctor. "And
from that," he said, "you can tell if I'm normal?"

"Normal?" Herbert Gray smiled ingenuously. "I've
never met a normal person in my life. Is a man who
wants to be president of the United States normal? Or
how about Mother Theresa? It's a meaningless word
in human terms. People relate to others well or they
don't, are productive or not, well adapted to who they
are or unhappy with who they are."

Carol felt that the psychiatrist had left Tommy's
question unanswered, probably on purpose. "But we
understood from Myra," she said, "that you'd be giving an opinion about whether . . . whether Tommy
could have done . . . these things . . ."

"Oh, that I can do."

"How?" Tommy asked.

"I put together a picture of a personality. On one
level it's quite crude. How well can I know you in three
hours? But on another level what I see is a whole range
of reactions, and that tells me how disturbed a person
is, how accurate their view of themselves and the
world is."

"Don't take offense," Tommy said, "but couldn't
you make a mistake?"

"About this?" Herbert Gray replied. "I don't think
so. Can I know if you'd return a ten-dollar bill to a
salesclerk who meant to give you a five? Maybe not.
But will I know if you're capable of committing a series
of savage homicides? Oh, yes, I'll know." Gray stood
up. "Miss Warren, Myra has told me how helpful
you've been to your brother, but today it's between
him and me. So, if you wouldn't mind . . ."

Carol rose, nodded at Tommy and gave him an encouraging smile. She followed the psychiatrist to the

small vestibule, where he held the outside door open for her. "Don't look so frightened," he said. "This isn't brain surgery, you know. It's only talk."

She thanked him and hurried up to the street. Heading for the crosstown bus stop on Central Park West, though, she couldn't help repeating in her mind the psychiatrist's last words. *Only talk,* he had said. As if talk were so harmless. How did the Deep Woods Killer begin the encounters that lured women to their deaths? With nothing more than that—only talk.

The Delmar Gardens nursing home, outside of Hewlett Harbor, felt like a small private club, not the bleak warehouse for old people that Carol had expected. Though a modern three-story building, it had been decked out with white clapboard siding, creating an atmosphere of home, not hospital. The expansive grounds, with clusters of trees and a small duck pond, had been landscaped to accommodate wheelchairs, with asphalt paths and waist-high railings.

"Nice, ain't it, sweetie?" Culley Nelson asked as they stood by the front door. "Pete wouldn't mind this."

Carol agreed. "I'm sure Tommy would approve, too."

"How is my boy?" Culley asked. "Works too damn hard, that kid, just like me and your dad."

Yes, Carol answered quickly, the business was absorbing all of Tommy's time these days.

"That's life," Culley said. "You work your butt off 'cause you don't know how to do anything else."

Carol followed him inside. In his search for a place that Pete wouldn't find oppressive, Culley told her, this one stood out head and shoulders above the rest.

At the end of the entrance hall they were met by Eli Garroway, the director. A portly man in his fifties with wavy gray hair, he gave them what he called his "tour of the ship." The place was spotless, the furniture in the lounges sturdy but comfortable Early American. The clinic included not only a full-time doctor, but also three nurses and a part-time pharmacist.

"You've come at a good time," Garroway said. "We try to keep the number of Alzheimer's patients to a minimum, they do need a lot of attention. But we have a spot open and we'd be glad to have Mr. Warren."

"It's a great relief," Carol said, and thanked him.

"Do walk around some more, if you like," Garroway said, "but if you could make a decision today, it would be very helpful. We can fill out some forms and set a date."

Culley took Carol's arm and they walked through the rear sun porch onto the back lawn.

"Culley, can Dad afford this? These places—even the snake pits—cost a fortune."

"Some of it's covered by Medicare, sweetie, and Pete's pension should figure in. With what you'll get for the house, you'll have a good-sized fund. But you know if you and Tom are short . . . well, I'm doing a good business these days."

"No, Culley—"

"You gonna tell me how to spend my money? The wife and I got lots more of it than we need."

Over the years Culley Nelson had helped the Warrens through hard times. He had paid for large chunks of Tommy's education and had often sent Carol unsolicited checks when she was starting out as a writer and illustrator. But she felt that he'd done more than enough.

"We can manage it," Carol said. "Though I might look for a place that's not so—"

"Sweetie, are we gonna put Pete somewhere he'll get depressed and mope around? I can't see that. And don't you think I know it ain't easy to take money? You can hurt a man if you do too much for him. I worried about it with your dad all the time, worried about it when Tom came to me for a loan for the business—"

"I didn't know he did that," Carol said.

"I told him to keep it under his hat. It's nobody's business but his and mine. Anyway, when you need, you take, that's all. So don't think about money now. This is a good place for Pete, and we'll all swing it."

It occurred to Carol that Delmar Gardens was not the kind of place to accept new residents on short notice. There had to be a waiting list. Yet Culley had said Dad could move in whenever Carol and Tommy decided the time had come.

"Culley, how did it happen that they'll take Dad so fast?"

"They had a vacancy, some guy died," Culley said, but the words came too fast.

"Is that right?" she said with obvious disbelief.

"Okay, so maybe I promised 'em a little donation. Is that a crime? Don't call the cops on me."

Relenting, Carol smiled and took Culley's hand. "You're a saint," she said.

"Not in this life," he said with a wry chuckle, "but in the next, who knows? Come on, let's fill out those forms. I want to visit Pete here and shoot some pool with him. And in a couple of years, maybe Sarah'll check in with me, and my kids'll visit, and you and Tom'll visit, and then you'll leave us doddering old coots and try to figure out what the hell life's about. And when you do, maybe you'll let me in on the big secret."

24 AT THE END OF THE CORRIDOR Myra Cantrell stood waiting outside her office, framed in the glow of a recessed light. "Dr. Gray's just arrived," she said as they approached. "I would have called you but I found out the results only ten minutes ago myself. I think you'll be pleased."

"Thank God," Carol said. She turned to Tommy. His face was expressionless, as if he'd been drugged. Even after she had put her arms around him, several seconds passed before he responded.

"I knew I wasn't crazy," he said finally, returning her embrace.

"Before we go in," Myra said, "there's something I wouldn't want to mention in front of Gray in the event he ever has to testify. I spoke with the New Jersey police this morning about pursuing Frank Matheson. They're not especially fond of taking direction from me . . . so we'll give them a day or two and then start pushing for action."

She swung the door open. On the couch sat Dr. Herbert Gray. He stood with his hand out, and as Carol shook it and watched Tommy do the same, she realized that Herbert Gray had not offered it yesterday—when Tommy had been a potential psychopath.

"Herbert," Myra said, "we're ready to hear your opinion."

The psychiatrist sat down. "Normally I would present my findings in writing," he said, "but I understand the urgency here." He reached into his briefcase and pulled out a manila folder, then turned to Tommy. "Mr. Warren, you shouldn't take it unkindly if I say that I see all sorts of problem areas in your life." Gray paused to look at his notes. "An occasional distancing from your emotions, and a touch of grandiosity that alternates with feeling low for no particular reason. Such characteristics are within the continuum that we call mental health, though you might find therapy useful at some point." He smiled slightly. "But whatever your problems, I'm thoroughly satisfied that you're utterly incapable of the bestial crimes you're accused of. There are a plethora of reasons for my judgment, and I'll put them in my written report, but for you the important thing now is that I'm fully prepared to testify on your behalf in any court."

The relief surged in Carol, but with it came resentment—at the police, at Paul Miller, at a system that could so uncaringly skew an ordinary person's life.

Myra Cantrell was smiling at Gray. "Well, that's very good news, Herbert. We all appreciate your doing this so quickly."

"That sure includes me," Tommy said gratefully.

"You see," Gray said, "being nervous wasn't fatal."

Tommy gave him an embarrassed grin and turned to Myra. "So how do I go on from here?" he asked.

From the look on Myra's face, Carol thought, the lawyer was savoring a great triumph. If Myra had never quite endorsed Tommy's innocence, she had still given her professional best to end the slanders against him.

"Over the next few days," Myra said, "I'll discreetly mention Herbert's judgment to a few people. Combined with the lineup and the lack of other evidence, I think we can get the New Jersey police to leave you alone. Once they back off, everybody else should follow suit. Of course the best thing," Myra added, "would be if the real killer could be caught."

"I just want my life back," Tommy said plaintively, "as much of it as I can salvage."

He meant Jill, Carol thought sadly. It was possible that Tommy had lost the only thing that really mattered to him. And perhaps only because he had tried to help one person—Frank Matheson.

"Dr. Gray," Carol asked, "if you can say what kind of person isn't capable of really awful . . . violence against women, do you have a way of knowing who *is* capable of it? What kind of person is the killer? What makes him who he is?"

Herbert Gray folded his arms on his chest and brooded on the question. "You're asking me to define the origins of the most complicated illness. Homicidal sexual psychopaths aren't easily understood. We could say that this man has a crippled sense of identity, so that he changes the way he relates to people the way you and I change clothes. We could say he probably had a highly charged relationship with his mother, with an element of manipulation by the mother that turned into a battle for control, and that as a consequence he has a deep-seated rage against women. I could speculate on all of those things, and yet, obviously, one rather major element would be missing."

The psychiatrist looked from Carol to Tommy to Myra.

"The missing element," he went on, "is a mystery. I could find ten men with identity problems who burned with rage toward women. Yet not one would be a psychopath who sought seismic sexual release through torture or violence. And even though the past defines who a person becomes, it's not always in ways we can see. Given the same parents and similar childhoods, two children will still grow up into entirely different adults. In the end, there simply may not be a clinical explanation for the existence of these human monsters." Gray paused and smiled in seeming bemusement before continuing with evident reluctance.

"I suppose as a doctor I shouldn't say this, it's what you'd hear from a priest—though even Freud wrote about the instinct for destruction and talked about it in terms of God and the Devil. So perhaps I wouldn't be too amiss if I tell you that the kind of crime we're dealing with may not lend itself to logical diagnosis. The truth may be that this kind of killer is nothing less than the embodiment of evil." Gray paused, as though the words were a revelation even to himself. "Pure evil."

The effects of the forensic psychiatric report met Myra's predictions. Already she had been in touch with the New Jersey police, and though officially Tommy would remain a suspect, they had backed off from any intention of making an arrest. On the other hand, there was little movement toward instituting a more thorough investigation of Frank Matheson. "We're sandbagged by police politics," Myra explained. "Matheson lives out of the Jersey jurisdiction. But the New York police have already run a check on him, and they say he looks clean. They'll want fresh evidence to reopen his file."

"Then what can we do?" Carol asked.

"I'm working on it," was all Myra could offer.

Carol realized that the situation was exactly the one Paul Miller had described—police departments covering their tracks, avoiding cooperation for political reasons, refusing to admit their own failures. What would happen, Carol wondered, if Frank Matheson got wind of the investigation? He would not only destroy evidence, she thought, but find new ways of shifting his guilt.

At one time Carol would have turned to Eric. But she could only think now that he was a policeman, committed by his job to pursuing one of the suspects on the police list. Once Carol had relied on a vague idea of cosmic fairness—some notion that the universe took care of good people and hurt the bad—but now, as she faced both monstrousness and unfairness beyond comprehension, those conventional faiths were gone. The system had done nothing to apprehend Frank Matheson, and as far as she could tell no one seemed inclined to change the situation.

25 FOR DINNER IN THE COUNTRY Frank had chosen The Box Tree, a restaurant north of the Westchester County border. He had lobbied for an early evening meal as more relaxing, and as a consequence Carol felt herself doomed to spending more time with him than she had hoped would be necessary.

Arranging the date had demanded more cunning than she had imagined she possessed. But after her conversation with Myra, Carol had decided that only by her own swift intervention might evidence against Frank be gathered. She had planned with great care how to reclaim Frank's good graces. A call to apologize for her temperamental outburst in the car after the lineup, then a plea for compassion embroidered with a hint of tears. If he could forgive her, she'd be forever grateful. He forgave her quickly enough that she was able to suggest a special date—an elegant meal in the country.

All the while she spoke to him on the phone, she had held in her mind a vision of his performance as the Little Tramp—with his baggy pants and bowler hat and cane . . . his blind man's cane.

Because he was returning to the city late in the day from a hospital appointment on Long Island, Frank had asked Carol if she could meet him at his apartment to save time. He had just been coming out of the building when she arrived. At first, distracted, he seemed not to recognize her, or even to expect her, and then came the smile spreading across his face. The change—from a disturbing look of irritation to a winning boyishness—froze her.

That was how he did it, she thought. He was a chameleon, able to transform himself into a helpless man with crutches, a blind man with a cane. *You're very good,* she thought, *but we'll see who's the better actor tonight.*

On the drive to the restaurant and all through the formalities of being led to the table and ordering the food, Carol struggled through inane conversation with him. While she made one innocuous remark after another, she wondered if he could see the terror churning inside her. What would he do if he guessed her motives?

Now, fastidiously sipping his wine and waiting for his dinner to arrive, Frank said, "What a great idea this was! This is a lot nicer than having dinner in the city."

"And you were the one," said Carol brightly, "who hated living in the suburbs."

"It's different if you have to live here," Frank said wryly. "It's a much nicer place to visit." He surveyed the room—antique wood tables set with hand-painted Wedgwood plates, creamy walls, vases of lilies and sprigs of heather. "This is beautiful, don't you think?"

"Lovely," Carol said. *You monster.* She half-listened to his disquisition on the room's gracious design, but the specific points escaped her completely. When he moved on to discussing city politics and—after the food was served—to his review of a Springsteen concert he'd attended, Carol assumed she was nodding in the right places, for he went on volubly. Try as she might to participate, however, Carol had only the dimmest notion of what either of them had said.

". . . rougher for Tom."

The mention of her brother's name grabbed Carol's full attention.

"Yes, it has," she said automatically.

"Everybody at Meditron is talking about it. Any hope the cops will leave him alone?"

You'd like to know, wouldn't you?

"He's still a suspect," she said, allowing herself to be more talkative, hoping to lure him into some revelation. "His lawyer believes the police will keep tabs on him until . . . well, until there's another victim and Tommy has an airtight alibi."

There was a silence. Her strength was fading, draining out of her like sand in an hourglass. How did she maintain the facade? She looked down at her half-eaten meal—the rosettes of potato, slices of beef. She felt she might retch if she took another bite. *Get ready,* said a voice inside her. Then slowly, naturally, she dabbed her napkin at her lips and began pushing her chair away from the table.

"Is it warm in here?" she said, standing. "I think I'd like to freshen my makeup."

The moment had come. One gesture at a time, she ordered herself, don't rush it. Reaching under the chair, she made a show of peering at the floor. Hmmmm, show mild consternation, she thought. *Where is that damn thing?* She lifted the edge of the tablecloth, stared underneath into the well. No, not down there. A moment to reconsider.

"Did I bring my purse in from the car?"

"I didn't notice," Frank said.

"Oh, hell, I'll be right back."

She rose, pushed her chair in, turned toward the door. How soon would he realize her mistake? One step, two, three . . . and then she heard his voice.

"The car's locked," he called after her, standing. "I'll get it for you."

"No, don't be silly. Just give me the keys, I'll go out and get it."

He rummaged in his jacket pockets and produced the keys, dangling from a small silver half-ring with little spheres at each end.

Give him a smile now. "Thanks," she said. "I'll be right back."

She kept herself to a leisurely stroll, nodding at the headwaiter as she passed, and went through the door with no particular urgency. Well done, she thought, especially appreciating her decision to walk away without asking for the keys. That could have been a tip-off.

Outside she moved unhurriedly. He might be behind her, watching from the door. Finally, rounding the corner of the building, she broke into a trot. Approaching the car she noted the license number: 378-ESG. Different from the number Lisa Birnbaum had reported, yet as Carol had suggested, if the 3 were seen as an 8 . . .

She unlocked the door on the passenger side, reached under the seat, and retrieved her purse, then set to examining the car. The glove compartment was locked. She opened it, found only a collection of Exxon maps—New York, New Jersey, and Connecticut. She pulled them out and unfolded them. All three were crisp, new, and unmarked.

As well they should be, she thought, if you wanted to get rid of evidence.

Kneeling, she peered under both front seats. On the driver's side a can of tennis balls was wedged up against the springs, a small snow scraper on the passenger's side. Useless, Carol thought as she closed and locked the door, worse than useless. She ran to the trunk and popped it open. A bulb in the wheel well automatically flashed on. In the cove beneath the light Carol saw three long white canes, each with a metal tip.

Canes for a blind man.

Under the canes the industrial matting appeared to be stained. Carol leaned down and on closer inspection saw that the gray fibers were clotted, flattened out, and the blotchy stain was a brownish red. . . .

She felt a chill rise up through her, as if she were

slowly, cell by cell, turning to stone. Move, her mind commanded. Don't stand here forever.

She slammed the lid down. The sound, like the report of a gun propelling a racer from the starting line, sent her running.

As she crossed the room toward him, she felt her legs on the verge of buckling. She grabbed for her chair and dropped into it.

Frank smiled. "You found your purse. . . ."

"Right on the seat where I left it," she said.

A waitress came alongside with a cart of desserts and recited the choices.

In the strawberry torte, Carol saw blood. In the bottle of cassis, she saw blood.

"Ma'am?"

"I'll have the chocolate mousse," Carol said rather than reveal her lack of appetite.

Frank took the hazelnut cheesecake. With the desserts served, Carol lowered her eyes to the plate in front of her. No force on earth could compel her to eat.

"You okay?" Frank asked. "You look a little pale."

"I am feeling a bit woozy," Carol said. "Doesn't it seem hot in here?"

"Not to me," Frank said.

"My throat was kind of raw this morning, maybe I'm coming down with the flu." She raised her napkin to her cheek. Her skin was damp.

Frank was a model of gentlemanly concern. When Carol asked to go home, he paid the check quickly and retrieved her coat. All the way back to the city—confined with him in the car—she kept seeing the cane in the trunk, the stain on the carpeting. And the illness she had feigned in the restaurant became real. She was so spent, so tired to her core, that with anyone else she might have slept.

But she fought now with all her remaining strength to stay awake.

He escorted her into the lobby, holding her arm as though she were an invalid. At the elevator she said, "Thank you, Frank, it was a nice evening. I think I'll just go up and climb into bed."

"Let me make you a pot of tea or something."

"No, I should go straight to bed. If it's the flu . . ."

Frank took a step backward. "What's with you, Carol?" His voice was edged with irritation. "You're doing some number on me. We've been out on three dates and every time it ends with the same brush-off. First you were upset about this Miller character, then you were tired, and now it's the flu. I thought there was something screwy when you called to apologize. Maybe it's crazy, but I feel . . . tricked, *used.*"

His hostility seemed to grow as he spoke. The chameleon again, she thought. "Frank, I'm sorry," she said, holding her finger on the elevator button. "I really don't feel well."

"I'll bet you don't," he said quietly. "You know what I think? I think you're a tease—a damn cock-teaser."

Her control slipped. "That's disgusting, don't talk to me like—"

"Why did you want to go out with me tonight?" he asked, raising his voice. "I thought you were up to something weird. What the hell do you want, what's this charade all about?"

The doorman had heard him shouting and came running across the lobby, carrying a small lead pipe that the building staff always kept behind the front desk.

"Sir, you're causing trouble," the doorman said. "I think you'd better leave."

"Oh, I'll leave," Frank said bitterly. "I'll be glad to get the hell out of here." He started away, then spun back to Carol. "Tell your brother how I treated you. Maybe Tom'll fire me, except it's not a real good time for that, is it?" He started out again, then paused for one more shot. "And don't forget to tell him how you treated *me.*"

She was still shaking when she entered her bedroom. For several minutes she couldn't even take off her coat. She just sat in the dark, trembling.

Eventually the digital counter on the answering machine caught her attention. Two calls. One might be Tommy. She leaned across to press the "play" button, then fell into a reclining position as she listened.

"Carol, it's Margot. I think Tom's wrong, we have to do something. So I'm going ahead. If I do the decorator thing, I can get into Matheson's apartment and have a look. I'll call you later."

Oh, God, there was no point in Margot's risking anything now. Carol grabbed for the phone to call the Jenners. At the same time came two beeps from the answering machine, hang-ups, then . . .

"Carol, this is Larry. Have you talked to Margot today? I haven't had a word from her since this morning. I thought perhaps she stopped at your place. Ring me back, will you?"

Carol's hand froze in midair. She put the receiver down. When had Margot called? This afternoon, surely. Carol thought she had checked the machine before she left for Frank's and the message counter had read zero.

But could it have been earlier? Perhaps she had ignored the machine? She often did when she was working, and today, thinking about Frank . . . She couldn't remember.

Though why should she be so alarmed? Before coming to meet her, Frank had been in Long Island, hadn't he? There would have been no chance to meet Margot, no chance to—

The phone rang. She snatched it up and gasped a hello.

"Carol, didn't you get my message?" It was Larry Jenner. "I've been waiting to hear if you talked to Margot today."

"Larry, I've been out since late afternoon and just got home. Margot left a message, too—"

"What was it?"

". . . about some plans we were making," she murmured guiltily.

"Carol, listen: Margot is missing. I've just been to the police."

"Oh, God, no," she said in a hush. Could Frank kill—and then go to dinner afterward? Wasn't that, after all, the profile of . . . of Woodsie: a man who kept smiling through the worst of nightmares.

"Carol," Larry persisted, "exactly what did Margot's message say?"

"No . . . no . . . ," she cried softly, feeling all the futility of the incantation as the awareness dawned of what Margot could have suffered. "Oh, Larry, what have I done?"

Larry Jenner sat on the bed and listened for a third time to the message on the machine.

"I must call the police again," he muttered. From his wallet he extracted a piece of paper, then dialed.

Carol paced around the bed. "Larry, I would never have suggested that she do it, I told her not to, Tommy told her not to."

"Carol dear, please shut up for a minute."

She listened while Larry tried to explain to a policeman where Margot had been. But he seemed to be encountering resistance, repeating the story over and over, telling them about Frank, that Margot had tried to play a trick on him. . . .

Larry slammed down the phone and bolted up.

"Damn bureaucrats!" he shouted. "Goddamn civil

servants! Yes sir, no sir, we'll investigate tomorrow, sir, officially missing is seventy-two hours, sir, I'm sure your wife's all right—holy Christ, these morons."

"Larry, where are the kids?"

"In their goddamn beds, that's where they are!"

He flung the bedroom door open and stormed out, down the hallway toward the living room.

"How could you?" he bellowed, turning on Carol as she followed him. "How could you allow her to do this?"

Carol shrunk back. "Larry, believe me, I would never have encouraged her—"

"Oh fuck!" he said, banging his fist against the wall. "Damn world-saver, that's what she is, with her mother-of-all-living complex, taking in the stray cats of the world."

Larry stopped, sighed, leaned against the foyer wall, and buried his head in his hands.

Carol huddled next to him, frantic. "She'll be all right, Larry. Margot's a survivor."

Larry pushed her away. "Something terrible has happened. She may be dead." He flung an arm out. "Damn you! You killed her!"

He stalked away, and before Carol could collect herself, she heard the front door close with an explosive slam. She was immobilized by guilt. Larry was right, it was her fault. It was for her sake that Margot had become involved, and whether or not she had pressed Margot to act, she hadn't objected to her plan strenuously enough to prevent it.

Let her be alive, please, God.

Convinced that there must be some hope, Carol hurried to the phone. The woman who answered at the task force said Detective Gaines was unreachable but referred Carol to his precinct. Carol asked for the man to whom Eric had introduced her—his boss, Elward Daley. But Daley was also unavailable.

Of course: it was night, they had all gone home.

"But my friend is missing," Carol said urgently. "I think the man you're all looking for is to blame." The woman replied that she would try to alert one of the investigators, but that was the best she could do right now.

Carol hung up. Refusing to be defeated, she called Eric's precinct. The policeman on duty said Eric was out of the city and would not return until tomorrow.

Carol stared out the window at the darkened city. Did no one care?

26 HEARING THE CHIME of her front door, Carol ran to answer it, assuming Larry had returned to repeal his damnation of her. Words of relief and gratitude were already forming on her lips as she swung the door open.

Paul Miller was planted squarely on the threshold, the bulk of his overcoated figure filling the frame.

Startled, she stood immobile, and in her instant of hesitation he lifted one arm, stiffly outstretched, so that the door was buttressed open.

"There are reports," he said, "that your friend Mrs. Jenner has disappeared."

"How did you find out?" Carol demanded sharply.

"Carol, I haven't spent so long working on this case without making a few connections among others involved. Some are policemen in this city."

Fleetingly she wondered if one might be Eric. Could they know each other, be manipulating her together? Nothing was what it seemed—or there could be no Deep Woods Killer.

Miller took his hat off. "May I come in? I'd like to talk to you about Mrs. Jenner, do whatever I can to help."

We can talk right here, she thought to say.

But whatever fury remained in her heart, she saw him also as a father—a man who had lost a daughter—and she stepped back to admit him. As Miller came through the door, Carol felt more than a retreat from the boundaries of suspicion and distrust she had been living with for so long. She had invited him across an emotional threshold as well, from adversary to ally.

In the entrance hall he slipped out of his coat, which led to a fumbling dance of courtesy. He had apparently intended to toss the coat on a chair, but she offered him a hanger and prevailed in the duties of a hostess, storing his coat in the closet before she guided him to the living room.

"I'm sorry to trouble you," he said, "but could I have a glass of water? I've been talking to a lot of people tonight, and my throat is sandpaper."

She thought it might be a hint. "I have other things to drink, if you'd prefer."

"No, thank you, Carol. Water will be fine."

She turned and stopped, suddenly doubting whether to let down her guard and leave him alone. But it was an old reflex. No reason to fear him now.

When she returned from the kitchen, he was on the sofa, balanced on the edge as he looked around, the pose of a man careful not to seem too quickly at home. He took the glass of ice water from her with a murmured "Thanks" and drank it down in a single draft.

Setting the empty glass on the coffee table, he asked, "What was Margot Jenner doing when she disappeared? I have a feeling you know."

She felt assaulted. He had virtually accused her of putting Margot in peril. "You don't waste any time," she said tightly.

"Should I? Your friend is missing. Every second might make the difference."

"Then you feel she *is* alive?"

He paused barely a second. "I think you'd better tell me whatever you know."

She had told him about Frank. Now he sat urgently forward, pressing every point—how long Frank had worked with Tommy, the kind of cane he had used for his Chaplin mime, the identical company cars.

"But it wasn't just those things," Carol said. "It's the closeness to Tommy. I almost never doubted that when I searched his car I'd find something, some clue to connect him—"

"His car? You've searched it?"

She nodded, appalled at her own admission, knowing it had been foolhardy to take it on alone, that the same bravado might have cost Margot her life.

"What did you find?" Miller pressed.

When she reported the three canes and the dark stain in the carpet lining the trunk, there was a long silence. Then Miller rose slowly from the couch, his face tautly set in an expression mingling regret and resolve. "Jesus," he whispered to himself, then raised his voice. "I even remember the name. Matheson. He was on one of the early lists, when there were a couple of hundred suspects." His tone changed, became edged with reproach. "Until he was dropped."

"Dropped? Why?"

Miller rubbed a hand across his forehead, then walked idly across the room toward Carol's drawing table. "I don't know. Somewhere along the line he must have been questioned—or a background check was done without his knowing—and he came up clean. He could have had a convincing alibi for one of the times a victim was known to have disappeared."

"But that would rule him out."

"Assuming the alibi was real." Miller had reached the slanted drawing table, and he was gazing down at the unfinished sketches shuffled together on its surface.

"Then you agree with me," Carol said solemnly. "You think Frank Matheson is the killer."

Miller seemed not to hear her. He had become absorbed in looking through her work, pushing aside one piece of paper to bare another—furtively, as if he expected Carol to object.

"They're quite wonderful," he said at last. "You have an extraordinary sense of fantasy."

As much as she enjoyed such approval, she was piqued that he could let himself be distracted. "About Frank . . . ," she prompted.

Miller looked up, and his gaze focused on her again. "To check on him you've had to play up to him. I wonder if he knew you and Mrs. Jenner were friends. Do you think he has any idea what you were doing?"

"At the end of the evening he did seem to wonder about me."

Miller grunted. "He must have had suspicions when Mrs. Jenner entered the picture. Something about her must have alerted him."

"And he killed her," Carol blurted.

Miller held her in a stony gaze for a moment, his mind clearly racing on beyond conversation. Abruptly he strode past her chair toward the foyer.

Carol followed him at once. "He did, didn't he?" she said, no longer really asking. "He murdered Margot."

Miller retrieved his overcoat from the closet.

"Answer me, Paul," Carol insisted.

"I think you know the answer."

"Are you going to Frank's?"

"No. Now that you've told Mrs. Jenner's husband, the police will visit Matheson—maybe tonight. But I doubt they'll find anything. There are other places I should get to before Matheson has a chance to cover his tracks." He had pulled Carol's lined trench coat from the closet, and now he held it out to her. "You're coming, too. I can't leave you here alone. You and Mrs. Jenner conspired, after all. Eliminating her wouldn't completely . . . solve the killer's problem."

Carol took her coat and slipped it on without protest. Wherever Miller led her now, she would follow.

*   *   *

For the first few minutes after they were in his station wagon, Miller made no conversation. It was well past midnight, and in the light traffic they made rapid progress driving west across town.

Miller explained his intention—to break into the Meditron offices and search past records on the use of company cars. Logs were often kept for each vehicle, the mileage, the purpose of long trips. Tommy himself had willingly turned over records relating to his own car, but nothing significant had been revealed. A similar check of Frank's records might be more fruitful. "The killer has covered a lot of territory, after all, moving from state to state. A pattern might show up."

It made sense, Carol thought. "But why break in? Tommy has keys. If we call him—"

"No," Miller said sharply. "For your brother's sake, we've got to keep him out of this. You don't want anyone to say he had a chance to tamper with evidence."

"Should we be alone, then?" she asked. "Or asking for help?"

Miller frowned. "We can't bring the police in. They'd need a search warrant for what we're after, and by the time it came through, the chance to get hard evidence might be lost." The possibility seemed to fire his anger anew, and he began muttering to himself. "Stupid . . . all this time wasted. If only I'd checked out Matheson myself before his name was cut from the list . . ."

"You've been on your own," Carol offered lamely. "You couldn't do everything."

"Except I've always known the damn police were skipping over things, not playing this tight enough. Matheson's alibis should have been double-checked." Stopped at a red light, he glanced at her bleakly. "If you'd come to me, Carol, if you could have trusted me. Then Mrs. Jenner at least—"

"Oh, Paul," she sighed miserably, "I see that now."

The outburst drew his eyes to her again. In a gesture

of regret at the pain he had caused her, he reached out and touched her arm. "Forgive me," he said. "I should know better than anyone how you get caught up, feel your only chance is to go it alone."

Carol smiled at him in the darkness and sat back. But as they were crossing Broadway, on their way to the George Washington Bridge, another idea about Frank occurred to her.

"Paul, the garage where Frank keeps his car is only a few blocks away. I went with him earlier tonight. If we could get into the trunk, take a piece of that carpet . . ."

"Where's the garage?" Miller said at once.

She couldn't recall which street, but she remembered a large orange neon sign running vertically down the side of the three-story building, with one letter darkened so that it read PA KING. It took only ten minutes of cruising before they found it on Eighty-fourth Street.

They sat in the car contemplating the front of the garage, a yawning entrance beyond which lay a gloomy interior lit by a dirty-bluish light. No cars entered or left.

"At this time of night," Miller observed finally, "business is bound to be slow." From the glove compartment he took a small black leather pouch, which he slipped into his coat pocket. Signaling Carol with a nod to join him, he got out of the car.

They paused at the edge of the entrance, scanning the maze of cars in tightly packed ranks. Pointing a finger, Miller indicated the wire-glass-paneled door of a small office near the rear. Through the glass, the screen of a small black-and-white television could be seen flickering, an attendant watching with his back to the door.

"Do you know where Frank's car is kept?" Miller said, his voice hushed.

Carol shook her head. "They delivered it on the

street. No, wait . . . they drove it up the ramp from the basement.''

As they scuttled quickly down the ramp opposite the attendant's cage, Carol's heart started to race, every beat thudding against her chest. The vaulted basement, with its low ceiling supported by massive pillars, was not so different from what she might draw as a dungeon in one of her fantasies. In the dim light the glass lenses of the headlights and taillights winked out from behind the pillars like the eyes of hostile animals.

As soon as they came down onto the level floor, Carol spotted Frank's car, parked between two pillars directly facing the ramp. At the sight of it she stopped. Miller, several feet ahead of her, spun around.

"You all right?"

She motioned to the car. "There it is."

"I know—just like Tommy's."

"Paul," she said, pointing, "the license plate."

Miller stared at it, swore softly. "A three and an eight," he said. "Close enough."

From his coat pocket he withdrew the leather pouch. He zipped it open and removed a thin metal shaft the length of a pencil, with a sharply pointed end attached to small flanges. He slipped it into the lock of the trunk compartment, gently waggled it from side to side, up and down. The lid popped open, and the interior light went on automatically.

The trunk was empty, the canes gone. Where there had been a large stain in the carpeting of the trunk, there was now an obscure patch that was only a faint shade darker.

"It's been cleaned," Carol said.

"If it was blood," Miller responded quietly, "it can't be completely washed away."

He replaced the jimmy in his pouch and took out a small flashlight, a pair of tweezers, a pair of blunt-tipped scissors, and a few plastic sandwich bags. Switching the flashlight on, he handed it to Carol and told her to direct it at the faded stain. Then with the scissors and tweezers he began collecting samples of carpet.

"Sweep the light around the corners," he instructed. As Carol moved the beam along the edges of the trunk, Miller reached out with the tweezers several times and plucked up small things—a scrap of paper, a shard of glass, a bit of dust—which he put into separate bags. At last he took the flashlight from her, replaced everything in the pouch, and pressed the trunk lid shut. With the task completed, Carol expected him to move quickly toward the ramp. Instead Miller remained in place, looking down thoughtfully.

"Christ," he said softly. "I hope to God we didn't just blow this case." Then he started away.

Carol hurried to stay alongside as they climbed the ramp. It seemed steeper on the way up. "How could we, Paul? If that was blood—"

Miller seemed to move effortlessly. "Carol, we had no legal right to enter that car. No matter what our samples prove, they'd probably be declared inadmissible evidence in a trial."

"Then what's the point?"

"For us to know the truth, the police to know."

They were at street level. The attendant in his cubicle remained immersed in his late-night movie as they exited to the sidewalk.

"But knowing won't be enough," Carol said. "He has to be stopped, punished, made to pay for what he's done."

In the middle of the street, as they were crossing to his station wagon, Miller suddenly halted, as if he had recalled something left behind. Slowly he turned, and in a gentle voice like one Carol might use to read to a child, he said, "Of course he'll be stopped, Carol. No matter what else happens, he will be punished."

*   *   *

The Meditron offices occupied space in one of several low, modern buildings that comprised an industrial park along Route 4 in New Jersey, a twenty-minute drive from the George Washington Bridge.

They traveled in silence again, but there was none of the tension Carol had felt earlier. She had joined Miller in his mission. As they rode across the bridge, she was caught by the long view of the Hudson River glimmering like a strand of blue silk under moonlight, its border stitched with the silhouettes of faraway skyscrapers. Her gaze drifted then to Miller's shadowy profile as he sat at the wheel. How queer it felt to be here with him. He had been her tormentor and pursuer, had seemed at times to be the general of a whole army arrayed against her—the man who wanted to condemn her brother. Yet now he seemed the best hope of saving him.

Music cut into her thoughts. Miller had turned on the radio. A Chopin nocturne played to its end, then the announcer came on and identified the station— WQXR. A kind of omen, Carol thought, evidence of a shared taste at the very moment in which the gap between them was closing. She almost remarked on it, but he spoke first.

"I've done things badly, Carol. I've . . . bedeviled you—that's the word, 'bedeviled.' All I can say is that I'm sorry. You're a special person, you didn't deserve—"

"It's all right," she cut in, surprisingly touched by his confession. "You had your reasons."

"Each step of the way," he went on, "I've done what I felt I had to do. But I never know when I've gone too far." He paused. Now on the radio a Mozart sonata was playing, and it soothed their silence. "This has been my life. Yes, I had my reasons. But are they good enough? Was I crazy to begin, I sometimes wonder, am I crazy to continue?"

Carol kept watching him but said nothing. He was talking for his own benefit, thinking aloud.

They had moved onto Route 4, six lanes that sliced through a cluttered, garish suburban sprawl of discount appliance stores, all-night diners, and gas stations. Brightly lighted signs cast a flickering glow on Miller's face as they passed by. The grim set of his features, Carol thought, looked more sad than vengeful.

"Sometimes," he continued, "when a few weeks went by and nothing new turned up, I asked myself if it wasn't time to quit. I even tried once. Stepped back into my business for a couple of days. But that was as long as it took before I knew it was too late. I couldn't think about those problems—burglar alarms for a suburban bank—while I knew this was going on, a madman taking one life after another, his relentless timetable, month by month another victim."

"Is it really like that?" Carol asked. "On a schedule?"

"There's a pattern with almost every serial killer. Why they start—what kicks off the impulse—nobody knows. But then it has to be satisfied again and again. It isn't always regular. At the start of the Deep Woods case—going back five years—there seemed to be one every three or four months. But the pace picked up. Six a year. Then twice as many. That's the pattern. The need to kill keeps building, and it's almost like a drug. The murderer gets a tolerance for it, and the only way to get the high is to have more, always more."

The sweet strains of the Mozart went on playing under Miller's lecture. Carol felt almost as though the music were defiled by what he had said. She reached over to switch it off.

Miller went on as if he hadn't noticed. "Of course, that makes it harder for him to maintain his pose of innocence. And eventually it's impossible, unbearable. With this killer it hasn't happened yet, but if we don't catch him soon, the need will overtake him, and he'll probably go into overdrive. He'll start picking victims indiscriminately, and then we'll find clues easier to come by."

It had already happened, Carol thought. With Margot.

"He's given you a chance now," Carol said. "To find things he might have been more careful to conceal."

"More of a chance than we ever had before," Miller allowed. "But we're not yet at the stage I'm talking about—when the killer feels himself getting hemmed in, and he loses control. A time when his impulses just . . . explode."

"What will he do then?" Carol asked shakily.

"Go on a rampage, probably," Miller replied. "Kill two or three women, one right after the other."

While Paul expertly jimmied a rear first-floor window of the darkened two-story building that housed the Meditron offices, Carol remained beside him, obediently performing as "lookout." He worked methodically, showing no fear of being discovered.

The window opened into a small maintenance room—a sink, mops leaning against the wall. Miller pushed the top pane inward, and the entire frame tilted to let him crawl through. He helped Carol in, then pushed it shut. She followed him out to a corridor, where she pointed toward the double doors at the end: the Meditron offices. Standing in the darkened hall, she was suddenly struck by the reality of what they had done—how strange it was to be here like this, breaking in.

"Paul," she whispered.

He stopped, turned.

"Paul, you broke into my apartment."

"No, Carol, when—"

"You're very good at this," she said. "Tell me the

truth. Did you go into my apartment looking for evidence against Tommy?"

He stared at her for a long moment. "No, Carol," he said firmly, "I didn't."

He went back to work, running his finger around the metal frame of the double doors. The building was silent except for a low clicking sound coming from the other end of the corridor. A brokerage firm, Carol remembered—it was the stock ticker. She followed as Paul stepped down the hall, back to the maintenance closet, and reached up to what looked like a fuse box high on the wall. He opened it, studied the interior for a moment, then with his fingers separated several strands of wire—red, blue, and black.

"Cheap security," he muttered. "If they'd used my outfit, we'd never have gotten in here." He took a knife from his pouch and cut the black wire.

At the Meditron office he took from his pouch a thin strip of plastic and inserted it between the two doors. Working a jimmy into the keyhole, he turned it once. The lock sprung, and the door opened.

The entry seemed so effortless that Carol wondered if the solution to a crime engaging hundreds of law enforcement officers over several years could be obtained so easily. But of course others hadn't known exactly where to look. Still, she had the odd sense that perhaps this was too easy, as if a lure had been cast, a trap laid.

They made their way along the central corridor of the suite with Paul sweeping the beam of his small flashlight across each room they passed. Wherever he saw banks of filing cabinets, he went to pull the drawers and riffle the contents. When they came to an office marked by a plaque etched with Frank's name, Carol was surprised that Paul didn't even bother to enter. She tugged at his sleeve and pointed to the name.

"No files in there," Miller said softly.

"But the desk, the cabinets—"

"There wouldn't be anything," Miller insisted. "What we came for, Carol—the only thing we can hope to find—is a piece of evidence that can't be hidden because it doesn't belong to Frank, because it's just a part of the company records and maybe he didn't fully realize how it could be used against him." He continued along the hallway and she trailed after him.

They checked through more than a dozen rooms before arriving at an office with several desks and the word ACCOUNTING on the plaque next to the door. Here Miller pulled several drawers open. When he paused over one, Carol saw in the bright beam of his light a collection of folders all marked on the edge with large tabs displaying the same words: "Travel, Logs and Expenses." Paul flipped one open, studied it a second, then replaced it and looked at another. He had opened the fourth folder when she noticed him straighten slightly.

"Jackpot," he said, staring at the sheets cradled in his hand. "This is it, Matheson's trip record." He pushed the file drawer shut and rolled the folder into his overcoat pocket.

"C'mon," he said urgently, "we can go home."

27

SHE OPENED HER EYES to see a pair of tall wrought-iron gates framed in the beam of the station wagon's headlights. Drowsy from the long ride, Carol rolled her head languidly toward Paul and saw him press a small button mounted below the dashboard. The massive gates parted and slid back, and the car drove through.

Home, he had said, explaining that he kept his records there—times and places for the disappearances of the victims. At first Carol had resisted accompanying him. But Margot's disappearance, he had reminded her, meant that Carol too was in jeopardy and shouldn't stay alone in the city.

"You can rest while we drive to my place in Westchester," he had said. "Trust me, you'll be safer this way."

But could this be his home? The long driveway ended at a circle of lawn in front of a house of gray stone, the station wagon's headlights sweeping over an imposing front portico and rows of curtained, darkened windows bordered by wood timbers. Only then did Carol realize what a huge, sprawling structure it was: not merely a house, but a grand mansion built in the Tudor style.

She recalled Paul's mention of having his own business, and money enough to support himself for years on his private quest. Any loving father, she had thought, could have been moved to search for his daughter's killer, even if it meant selling his last possessions to stake himself. Yet if this was Paul's home, there was little question that he was a man of some wealth. Thinking back, Carol realized that there had been subtle hints of affluence. There was the way he dressed, almost a fashion for another time, a style that marked him as standing apart from the crowd. And there had been his large family, too—not in itself a sign of wealth, but coupled with the love of books he'd imparted to his children, it pointed to the sort of cultured upbringing that money made possible.

As if Paul thought she might still be asleep, he got out of the car quietly and eased the door closed before walking around to open the passenger door. Carol followed him silently to the house, carrying the files that had been in her lap as she dozed.

"This is where you live?" she couldn't help asking.

"When I live anywhere," he replied, unlocking a lacquered front door lit by two carriage lanterns.

Inside, he flipped a bank of switches, throwing light from a chandelier onto a soaring two-story entrance hall furnished in a manner suitable to the grand exterior—a heavy Gothic credenza, high-backed chairs with maroon cushions, an ornately carved table. Adorning the credenza was a crystal vase holding an elaborate arrangement of dried flowers, and on the wall above it, facing a wide stairway, hung an immense Chinese tapestry.

Crossing to an archway at the left, Paul turned more switches, illuminating a large living room. Here the decor was much less severe, with a soft couch and chairs arranged around a fireplace, all in muted colors. It was a comfortable room, yet there was a curious faded quality to everything. Carol felt that it hadn't been a family's gathering place for a long time.

It had not, however, gone completely unused. The living room was evidently where Paul worked on his investigation. In front of the floor-to-ceiling French windows, a long refectory table had been positioned—

hastily, to judge from the way other pieces of furniture
were pushed around either end of it. Shoved beneath
the table were several cardboard boxes, and the surface was covered with stacks of dossiers, photographs,
and news clippings. At one end sat a telephone surrounded by pens and pencils. On a broad stretch of
wall between the windows, several maps had been
taped up.

Removing his hat and coat, Paul tossed them on an
easy chair, then crouched to one of the cardboard
boxes under the table and pulled out several files.
Standing, he reached out for the folders Carol was
holding.

"Let's see how those travel logs match up."

Carol glanced to the phone. "Paul, before anything
else, could you see if the police have news about Margot?"

"Yes, of course. I should have thought of it." When
he dialed without checking a directory, Carol was reminded that he had spoken of having his own police
contacts.

He spoke to someone in a grim monotone for only
a couple of minutes before hanging up. "No sign of
Mrs. Jenner. They brought Matheson in and couldn't
get a thing. He cooperated fully, answered every question. They had to let him go."

"But Margot was *there*, in his apartment."

"She was seen leaving the building." Carol started
to speak, but he was ahead of her. "Yes, he could have
waited for her outside, tracked her; there's no proof
he didn't. Trouble is, Carol, there's no proof he did."
Paul turned back to the folders on the table. "We've
got to hope there's something in here." He opened
the files and started laying out their contents, comparing them with the ones he had taken from Meditron.
Oblivious to Carol, he pored over his papers, scrib-
bling notes, occasionally moving to check a location

on one of the maps. Rather than slow him down, she let him work without asking for explanations.

Feeling the weight of sleeplessness, she drifted to the couch and lay down. Through half-closed eyes she gazed at the furniture, a grand piano at the far end, several oil paintings on the walls faintly visible in the dim light. She could imagine children once playing here, gathered around a holiday fire. Yet the room seemed sad and soulless now—and not only because Paul was using it for his work. The presence of his papers was, in fact, a touch of life. But something was off-key, Carol thought, something was missing. . . .

"Here's a break!" Paul erupted suddenly.

Carol looked around and saw him standing in front of a map, holding a sheaf of pages at eye level. "I've been comparing Frank's trips with dates and locations of the victims' disappearances, and there are three instances when he was much closer to the scene than your brother."

Carol hurried across the room. "Then you've got what you need?"

"It's a beginning." He tossed the papers onto the table. "Each time a victim was taken, the killer might have chosen the place precisely because it created an ambiguity. Frank and Tommy had to be aware of each other's day-to-day business. So Frank could have used your brother as a cover, fudged his own culpability by picking times that also put Tommy just as close to the scene."

"But the murders happened in four states," Carol said. "There have to be times when Frank could have been there but Tommy couldn't."

"I haven't found it yet," he said. In a harder tone he added, "But I will." His eyes locked with hers—as though he wanted to impress upon her that his vow had been made more for her than himself.

From somewhere in the distant recesses of the house came the resonant sound of a clock chiming

three times. Only then did Carol realize how tired she
remained, depleted by the constant call on her emotions of frantic worry about Tommy—and now, Margot. Was Larry right? Was it her fault . . . ?

"It's been a long night," Paul said at last. "I'm going
to stay with this awhile, but let me show you to a
room."

She nodded acceptance, thinking how strange it was
to put herself into his care, and yet moved by his sensi-
tivity to her need. She followed him to the second
floor. Passing the open doorways of shadowy rooms,
she glanced in and saw the outlines of unused beds.
How long since anyone else had lived here?

By a room at the end of the corridor, Paul stopped
and reached in to turn on a light. "I hope you'll be
comfortable," he said, then waited for her to look in,
as though she were a hotel guest whose approval was
required.

She was too tired to care where she slept, but when
she stepped into the room, she was held by its charm.
The walls were papered with a delicate floral pattern,
matched in the curtains and an upholstered chaise.
The fireplace had the sort of marble mantel that might
have come from an English country house, and the
bed was an antique four-poster with polished rails and
spindles.

"It's beautiful," Carol said.

Paul smiled. "I think you'll even find some nightgowns in there." He pointed to a dresser, then to a
closed door at one side. "And that's the bathroom."

When she thanked him, there was another moment
in which they stared at each other. He felt the strange-
ness of it, too, she knew—their metamorphosis from
enemies with opposing goals to . . . to what?

"Good night, Carol," he said, and before she could
answer, the door shut softly and she was left alone.

She went into the bathroom, took off her clothes,
and tiredly hung them on a hook on the back of the

door. She paused for a moment then, appreciating the
bathroom itself, with walls and floors of rose-tinted
marble. As she started washing her face with a bar of
perfumed soap, she thought of how loving a presence
had been at work here. And when she pulled a pink
bathtowel from the rack, she was struck by its softness
and the fragrance from a recent washing.

With the towel wrapped around her body she went
back into the room. Opening the top dresser drawer,
she saw the nightgowns. Whose were they? His wife's
perhaps. It would be too strange to wear one. As she
moved toward the bed, she noticed a pile of fashion
magazines on a small table by the chaise, then the
dressing table crowded with bottles of perfume and
makeup.

Did someone still live in this room? It was then that
Carol registered the two framed pictures on the dressing table. She went closer to inspect them, a group
photograph of a girl's-school field-hockey team, and
a black-and-white close-up of an attractive young
woman smiling directly into the camera, the sort of
frozen pose of hope that might appear in a college
yearbook.

It took only a second before she remembered seeing
the same picture once before—tacked to a wall in the
office of the task force.

With no less anguish than if it had been one of the
gruesome crime-scene shots, she whirled away from
the smiling face of Paul Miller's daughter, Suzanne,
and stood shivering for a minute, her head bowed, her
eyes squeezed shut.

There were no words to her prayer, but she knew
what it was and when it was done. Then she pulled
back the bedspread to reveal finely embroidered
sheets, turned out the overhead light, and found her
way back to the refuge of the bed.

*   *   *

In this fantasy she could not control the characters. Dana ran from trees that reached to strangle her with spindly-fingered branches, stumbled just ahead of sharp-toothed beasts, and slipped at last into a pit of red ooze that rose up over her chest and shoulders, until she was drowning. She called out for help, and then a handsome prince came, riding on a snow-white animal. The ooze seemed to thicken as it climbed up over her mouth, but she could see her rescuer moving toward her. She was cheering him on until she saw the sword in his hand on which a head was already impaled, a head with many faces all at once—Anne's, Margot's, the girl in the picture on the dresser. The red slime was rising, and she knew there was only one last breath in her. It came as a scream for help, a shriek loud enough to waken the gods who slept in even the farthest recesses of heaven.

And she was heard. A miraculous light shone down, and in an instant the bloody mire had receded, and she was safe.

Carol woke.

The lamp on a nighttable was on, and Paul was sitting on the edge of the bed, wearing pajamas and a red plaid bathrobe. She was trembling, fighting for breath.

"It's all right now," he said. "Just a bad dream."

But as though fearing she might slip down again into the bottomless slough of doom, she bolted up and threw her arms around him. For a moment she held on tightly, grateful for the solidity of his body, the feel of his woolen bathrobe against her skin anchoring her in reality.

"Hold me," she whispered desperately. "Oh, please, hold me. . . ."

Slowly his arms went around her, and she felt his hand move to her head and gently caress her hair. "Okay, Carol," he murmured. "It's okay."

She clung to him until her hysteria waned. Finally his hold loosened. "Better now?" he asked.

She nodded. And again she could neither speak nor pull her eyes from his. Having been transported with him, by him, on so many journeys of doubt, she saw him now in all his purity, a man of absolute dedication to the memory of a lost daughter. A man who had sacrificed everything else to fulfill his need. An impulse sent her hand to his face, and she slid it along his cheek.

He turned his head very slightly, not denying her, yet making the offer of denial. But she moved her hand behind his neck and gently urged him forward. Was it curiosity—or desire? She wasn't sure, but she wanted very much to feel his kiss.

Very slowly, deliberately, he lowered his head, put his lips on hers. He rushed nothing, kept his mouth lightly against hers, but she felt the heat flooding her body. Beneath the blanket she arched up toward him.

He pulled away. "Carol," he said simply—but in a tone of protest, even of warning.

But she held his arm. "Please, no, I don't want to be alone now."

He paused for a long moment, then reached over and turned out the light. In a moment he was naked beside her, kissing her again, his mouth moving then over her breasts, and coming back to her lips. His every touch was gentle, lingering, patient, giving.

And the wealth of his caring, too, seemed somehow to come as no surprise.

He was not beside her.

Opening her eyes to the morning light, Carol lay still, looking at the nearly bare trees outside the window, remembering his touch, and she reflected on the welling of desire that had invited his intimacy. Was it from a need for protection more than anything else?

Or merely a moment of weakness, an utter collapse of will, after being battered by so much uncertainty?

She rose and showered and dressed, her mind occupied all the time with the same questions, yet almost unconcerned with the answers. What was done was done, no regrets. Only time would tell if it was an aberrant moment . . . or if Paul Miller would stay in her life.

On her way to the stairs she glanced again through the doorways lining the corridor. In bright daylight none of the other rooms was marked by the personality or charm of his daughter's. Drab fabrics, no pictures on the walls. She recalled that Suzanne had been the only girl; Paul's other three children were boys. Perhaps they had been given more spartan treatment.

When she looked into the last room before reaching the stairs, she realized it must be Paul's. His plaid bathrobe and pajamas lay on an unmade king-size bed with a mahogany captain's chest at its foot. A handsome desk of the same wood occupied a niche by a window. Carol's eye was caught by two books sitting side by side on the desktop, their colored covers radiant in a stream of bright morning sunlight.

Whatever guilt she felt at entering his private domain was balanced by the memory of last night, the special grant that came with physical intimacy. The books on the desk, like the *Mother Goose* he had sent her, were also children's books, old and somewhat soiled. Turning them over, she found the same foil sticker affixed to the back showing that they had been purchased at The Bookworm. One was a finely printed edition of *Grimms' Fairy Tales,* the other A. A. Milne's *Winnie the Pooh* with the original illustrations of Ernest Shepard. Carol picked up the *Pooh* and leafed through it. Glancing over Shepard's gently whimsical illustrations of the bear and his friends, Carol wondered if she would ever be able to draw like this. How much had she been hardened by the ugliness that had invaded her life in the past few weeks?

She had come to the last picture and was about to put the book down when she noticed a loose page stuck in at the end. Had it torn free from the old binding while she was turning the pages? Flipping to the back, she saw with relief that it was a sheet of lined looseleaf paper, apparently an old exercise done by Paul's daughter. On every line the child's name was written in the same laboriously curlicued script that had appeared at the front of the *Mother Goose*. The only variation was on the top line where the girl had started by writing "Susanne," until she had realized the mistake—pointed out by a parent perhaps—so that the name was crossed out and written alongside with the correct spelling. "Suzanne with a 'z,' " Miller had said the first time she had seen him. Sure that the scrawled evidence of his daughter's childhood must be a treasured memento, Carol flattened it carefully into the back of the book. Laying the book down, she took in the other things on Paul's desk, clues to the man. A large green blotter in a black morocco frame, gold-handled scissors and letter opener in a case of black leather matching the blotter's, a calendar bordered in the same leather. An executive's desk.

Looking at the desk set, she remembered that one Christmas she had seen something similar at Mark Cross, considered it as a gift for Richard. In the end she had passed it up as too expensive—but what she recalled now was that the set had also included a matching picture frame. The absence of one on Miller's desk shouldn't have seemed remarkable—such sets were sold in all kinds of combinations—except it made clear a perception that had bothered her only vaguely until now. There were *no* family photographs anywhere in the house, none except for those of Suzanne in her room.

This was what had bothered her last night, she realized now, when she had sensed something odd about the room downstairs. No photographs. She had never been in a house of this size, the one-time home of a large family, without encountering evidence of their shared lives, pictures of vacations, of the children at early ages. So why not here?

Another of his lies?

No, she knew from the bookseller, Lumley, that Paul Miller had fathered several children.

Yet why did the house seem so barren of the events and memories that filled a family's history?

When she descended the stairs, he was standing at the long table in the living room, sifting through his files. A mug of steaming coffee sat near his elbow. As she entered the room, he looked around. He was wearing faded blue jeans with a pale tan cardigan over a blue striped shirt, and his graying sandy hair hadn't yet been brushed, so that wisps of it trailed over his forehead and stuck out here and there, lit up like fine copper wires by the sunlight behind him. Freed from the formal clothes that usually cloaked him like heavy armor, he looked years younger.

She hung back. Who was he?

When he held out a hand to her, the sort of gesture which, in past times, had accompanied a gentleman's request for a waltz with a lady, she found herself wondering only how to keep clear of him. How could she get away without creating a confrontation?

"Been at it a long time?" she said.

He moved toward her. "I feel as though I should ask your forgiveness."

She stopped abruptly and held her hands up, denying him the right to come any closer. "No, Paul. It was my fault, too. I wanted . . . that closeness. I haven't been . . . for a long time there hasn't been anyone, and I guess . . ." Her voice died, and he waited until she found it again. "With all this—the inhumanity that's part of it—I needed to believe there was something else. I don't know if it was more than that. I don't know if it matters. I'll never feel it was wrong . . . but now, I . . ." She trailed off.

"I see," he said very quietly. Squaring his shoulders, he added, "Whatever comes after this, I hope you'll never doubt how beautiful and special I think you are, how precious it was for me to be with you."

She nodded, trying not to do it curtly, but wishing this kind of conversation could end.

Paul took the cue. Turning back to his worktable, he said, "I checked with the police. No word yet." As if to distract her from brooding, he pointed to his papers. "But I've made some progress here. Two more cases where Frank's trips put him at least as close as Tommy to the disappearances, and several occasions when Frank is logged as having used Tommy's car."

"How could they let him go last night?"

"You can't charge a man without evidence, Carol."

"So a murderer stays on the loose."

"Not for the first time. It's what happens with serial killers. They're brought in as part of a police sweep, but they're let off because they pass muster."

Carol's shoulders slumped. She was anxious to leave now, to get home. But before she could say anything, Miller went on:

"I want to go to New Jersey and get this new stuff in the hands of the state police. But first, let me get you some breakfast." He started away.

"Never mind, I ought to be getting back to the city."

But he was out of the room, calling back that coffee was already made.

Waiting anxiously, she stood by the table where he worked. Still looking for hints to the truth about Paul Miller, she scanned his collection of paper, maps, reports, pictures. Why did he really immerse himself in the hunt? To avenge his daughter? And for the sake of that had he cut himself off from the rest of his family?

There was a stool by the table and she sat to await Miller's return. It was then she noticed that one of the cardboard file boxes under the table had been pulled forward and left open. He must have been using some papers from it. As her gaze hovered over the box, she saw some newspaper clippings, folded so the headlines were prominent. Carol tried to read them, then realized that the language wasn't English. Curious, she knelt and pulled the clippings out for a closer look. They were all in German, papers from several cities— Berlin, Frankfurt, Stuttgart. Several showed photographs of women arranged in long rows, and all had the same picture of a tall young man, with his head down, flanked by uniformed men who Carol supposed must be German police.

So other countries also had their serial killers. It was a testament to Miller's thoroughness that he would study a foreign case, too.

He returned carrying a tray with a plate of toasted English muffins and a cup of coffee. Eager as she was to go, she pretended to accept the food gratefully. While she nibbled, Miller gathered up the notes he wanted to bring to the police. Then he went upstairs, explaining that he wanted to change before going into the city.

He came to fetch her from the living room—looking, in all senses, like his old self: the suit and tie, the overcoat over his arm, homburg in hand.

When they were at the door, she turned back for a last glance at the house. How strange it was that she had come here, she thought, how strange the things that had happened. But it was behind her now. She knew she would never visit this place again.

The leave-taking at her apartment house was strained—as the ride had been. Paul tried repeatedly to draw her out, but in the wake of their night together Carol felt too compromised—even too ashamed—to bring up her doubts, and to open herself anew to his lies. The absence of family pictures except for those of his murdered daughter couldn't be mere accident. What secrets did he have to keep?

"Carol," he said, after coming around to open the passenger door, "I wish you could tell me what's wrong. If it's because of last night—"

She kept her eyes down. "It's not, Paul, so don't blame yourself. I'm a big girl."

"It sounds like you're sorry."

She lifted her eyes and found his. "I trusted you," she said quietly. "In spite of everything else, I let myself trust you. Tell me, Paul, was I right to do that? Answer just that one question. Did you deserve my trust?"

He held her gaze unflinchingly. Yet deep in the dark center of self revealed by the glint of his eyes, she saw the silent answer—echoed by the silence of his hesitation. She spun away, but he grabbed her arm.

"Carol. You don't always get to know right or wrong by answering just one question. There are other considerations. I thought . . . we were looking for the same thing."

The same thing? His phrase hung in the air as she hurried away into her building, afraid to ask any more questions, afraid to hear the answers. Her needs and wants, she had to believe, could not be the same as his.

28 "OH, MISS WARREN," the doorman said as she rushed in, "a couple of men were here asking for you—one of them left a card." Handing her the card, he lowered his voice. "Cops," he said confidentially. "Also, this package came for you a little while ago." From the counter below the house switchboard he retrieved a large manila envelope. The contents felt like a book. From Binny?

For a moment she thought the calling card was Eric's. At the right lower corner was the New York police shield she had seen on his card, but stamped across the center was "Gregory Kavana, Captain of Detectives." At the bottom were a few scribbled words: "Call as soon as you get in."

When she entered her apartment, she went to the phone by her drawing table but then pulled up short. What did the police want with her? To tell her Margot's body had been found? She couldn't bear to hear Margot pronounced dead. A minute of peace, she told herself, that was all she needed.

She put her coat away, then picked up the manila envelope. The book she found inside was one of her own, *Dana's Dark Ocean*, and clipped to the jacket was a handwritten letter. She only had to take in the first lines—written in a hasty scrawl with no salutation—to know whom it was from. Already realizing it might constitute evidence, she walked back to the phone as she read:

I'm sorry for you, Carol, if you think what you've told the police about me is the only way to save Tommy. I keep telling myself the strain of what you're going through must have pushed you off the deep end. How could you think I killed your friend Mrs. Jenner? I even bought another one of your books to see if it might give me a clue to what goes on in your head. I'd like to be able to forgive you. But I can't, I don't understand how you could do this to me, and when I look at your monster stories now I begin to see that maybe you could do this kind of thing—believe what you do about me—because somehow you're not normal. And so now I don't want the book . . . and I don't want you.

                                                    Frank

Carol's hand shook as she read the letter a second time, picking the phrases apart in her mind as though trying to decipher a code. Was there any unconscious giveaway . . . ?

She picked up the phone and dialed—Eric's number. If she had to deal with the police, let it not be with total strangers.

Thank God for small favors, she thought when she was put through to the detectives' squad room, and the man who answered said that Lieutenant Gaines was there and shouted for him to pick up the phone. A second later he came on.

"Gaines."

"Eric—"

"Carol," he cut in instantly, "are you okay? I wish I'd been here to help you, but I took Doug camping. I heard about your friend."

"What did you hear?" she asked anxiously.

"That she's missing. I've been told the police are trying to reach you for a statement. Where have you been?"

"With—" The truth caught in her throat. She couldn't let Eric know she had spent the night with Paul Miller. "—my father," she said, the safest lie that came to mind.

Eric didn't even challenge the story. He accepted as reasonable that, for one night, she might need a place to hide from the horror of losing Margot, from a killer. "Carol, hard as it is, we do need a statement—anything you can tell us about what Margot was doing when she disappeared."

Of course, she meant to say, she would do whatever was required. But at the mention of Margot a fresh wave of grief and guilt overtook her. She was filled with remorse, too, for the choice she had made last night. Her control slipped away, her voice breaking as she forced out an answer. "I can't face it, Eric, I can't face any more of it."

There was a momentary pause. "All right, listen— I'll take your statement, you won't have to deal with cops you don't know. I have to head over to the task force office. Meet me there in an hour. Will that be all right?"

"Okay," she answered softly. She wanted to tell him about the evidence in Frank's trunk, the note he had left her, and the travel records she had found with Paul. But before she could speak again, Eric had hung up.

She lowered the receiver into the cradle, stared at the book and the strange note from Frank. She realized that here, in her private refuge, she had lost her sense of feeling protected. Instead she felt the walls closing in on her, as if a riot were going on in the streets and the safety and quiet around her were only a delusion.

Snatching up the phone again, she called Tommy's home number. She needed desperately to connect, to know he hadn't been taken away from her—

He answered in a sleepy murmur on the fifth ring,

but forced himself awake as soon as he heard her voice. "I tried to get you before," he said. "Why aren't you answering the phone?"

She could no more tell Tommy about Paul Miller than she could Eric. "I needed rest," she said, "so I turned the bell off."

"Any word on Margot?" he asked.

Carol was stunned. "So you've heard . . . ?"

"Of course," he said wearily. "The cops woke me up at six o'clock this morning to question me about it."

"It's Frank again, Tommy." She told him now about the new evidence—Frank's travel log. "Paul Miller got hold of it."

"How?"

"I don't know," she said quietly. Was it the first time she had lied to Tommy? She hurried on. "But he told me it shows that Frank was near the places where victims disappeared—as near as you were. Miller's bringing the records to the police."

Her brother's silence cast an almost palpable chill. Then she heard him mutter, "That sonofabitch. He must have broken into our office."

"Does that matter, Tommy? He wants to help you."

"You really believe he wants to prove my innocence?"

"He said he was taking those records to the police," she repeated. "I'll check to make sure they got there."

Tommy said he'd tell Myra to check, too.

"Have you talked to Jill?" Carol asked.

Tommy drew a deep breath before replying that he had reached Jill's parents in Vermont. "Jill wouldn't come to the phone, though. Her dad said she's afraid of me."

"Maybe you should go up there and try to see her," Carol suggested. "Don't give up, Tommy. Show her she's wrong to be afraid."

"You know, I was thinking of that myself. I'll be

damned if I'll just throw in the towel and let her write me off. I may just go today."

Carol reminded him that they had planned to spend this afternoon with their father, moving him into the nursing home. "If you want me to handle it alone—" she started to offer.

"Could you? Every day that passes, I feel Jill can pull farther away."

"Sure, Tommy. Go see her. The way Dad is now . . . I hate to say it, but he may not even notice whether you're there."

Tommy sighed. "I know it's crazy, but yesterday I was thinking it's almost biblical—so many bad things at once, the trials of Job. But if this is supposed to make me stronger, teach me something, then God's making a terrible mistake. It isn't working."

There was a problem, Carol remembered—the appraisers were scheduled to assess the contents of the house for auction. Their arrival had been postponed so that Pete Warren wouldn't spend any time alone in empty rooms. "They're coming late tomorrow. If you want anything, I should mark it so it doesn't get sold."

There was nothing he really cared about, Tommy said, aside from childhood mementos still in his old room and stored in some boxes in the basement. "I figure a little family history might be interesting to have someday," he said. "That is, if I have kids."

It tore at Carol's heart.

"Are you sure that dumping this on you is really okay?" Tommy asked again.

Going to win Jill back, Carol insisted, was the most important thing he could do. "When this is all behind you, Tommy, Jill and the baby will make all the difference in getting life back to normal."

The large front room of the task force was noisier and more crowded than on her first visit. There seemed to be twice as many shirtsleeved men gathered around paper-littered desks, twice as many styrofoam coffee cups strewn around computers, and twice as much noise and smoke in the air. Carol imagined for a second that there had been a break in the case. She stopped at the center of the room, scanned across the groups of people talking.

She realized then that it was all happening because there was a new victim.

She felt a light touch on her arm and turned to see Eric at her side. He looked searchingly at her. "You all right?"

"Holding up," she said, and glanced around. "This is all about Margot, isn't it?"

He nodded grimly.

"Any hope?" she asked.

"We have more to work with than usual," he replied.

"Why isn't Frank Matheson under arrest?"

"Carol, honey, you may not like it, and I may not like it, but sometimes the system—"

"The system!" she cut in. "What about the blood in his trunk, the cane?"

Eric took a step back. "How do you know about that?"

"Paul Miller told me," she lied.

"Matheson has explanations," Eric said. "The canes had something to do with volunteer work for the blind."

"And the blood?" Carol asked. "First it's there, and then he washes it away a couple of hours later."

"He claims a piece of blood-testing equipment broke in transit and that it was the regular night for his garage to clean his car."

"Damn it," Carol cried, "you're letting him off too easy."

"Listen, it's not impossible," Eric answered calmly. "Like your brother, Matheson is in the business of supplying hospital equipment." He edged away. "I'll take your statement in a while, but first I—"

"There's something else that might help," Carol said quickly. She pulled Frank's note from her pocket. "This came to my house."

Eric took the note and ran his eyes across it. "We've got a guy who analyzes stuff like this. I'll see what he thinks."

"What do *you* think of it?" Carol demanded impatiently.

Eric shrugged. "It's weird. Either he's a guy who's pissed because he cared about you, and you turned on him, or—" *

"Turned?" Carol repeated in dismay. "Frank set things up to throw blame on Tommy. I've seen the proof."

Eric peered at her. "What proof?"

She told him about the travel logs Miller had obtained, and when Eric demanded to know where Miller had gotten them, she confessed to being with him when they broke into the Meditron offices.

"Broke in?" Eric muttered, pushing clawed fingers through his hair. "Carol, you've got to stay out of this—for your brother's good. That evidence is compromised now. We may not be able to use it."

"But the records show—"

Eric's thoughts were speeding down their own track. "Where are they now?" he broke in.

"Miller said he was taking them to the New Jersey police. He thought that would help Tommy most, because of the Fairleigh Dickinson case."

"All right," Eric said briskly. "Let me follow it up and I'll be back in a few minutes. Just sit tight." He hurried off down the corridor.

Carol went to the lounge. After running a stream of black coffee from the large urn into a styrofoam cup, she made an effort to sit patiently. But as other people hurried in and out, and she listened to the buzzing energy drifting in through the door, the tension became intolerable. Finally she got up and stepped back into the corridor.

Her intention had simply been to roam, but as she left the lounge, she found herself staring through the doorway into the room where the pictures of the victims were pinned up on a board. Her eyes rested on the array for a moment, seeing little more than a design, a morbid checkerboard of photographs, lines of faces laid out on a white background.

Suddenly her heart lurched, and the cup of hot coffee plummeted from her hand to the floor. There, at the end of one line, was a color photograph of Margot, standing in her favorite black silk dress, her face lit by one of her winsome smiles. Carol moved toward the maps and photographs as if drawn by a magnet. She knew exactly where the picture of Margot had been taken—at a party to celebrate Larry's last promotion. She and Margot had stood with their arms around each other as some guest had taken a flash snapshot. Along one edge of the print tacked to the board was an uneven line, where a scissors had excised the part that showed Carol. Larry must have provided the photograph. And was it also Larry, Carol wondered, who had cut it in half, his rage at her so great that he could no longer bear to see her linked to his wife even in a picture?

Carol brought her hand up over her eyes and rubbed at them, unable to face the pain of seeing Margot cataloged as just another victim. But in that moment of private darkness she still couldn't hide, for she was reminded of another picture, saw it looming in her mind's eye—Miller's daughter, the photograph she had seen in his house. Suzanne-with-a-z.

All at once the name and the phrase brought something else to mind: the piece of paper that had fluttered out of the book on Paul Miller's desk.

Carol's eyes flared open—and what she saw was

more in memory than on the board in front of her. *Suzanne-with-a-z!* Miller had always made such a point of how the name was spelled. Yet where she had seen it written, again and again, it had been misspelled once at the top as "Susanne." From the look of the handwriting, Carol had assumed the child herself was setting down her own name, doing an exercise.

But would a child misspell her own name? Even though it was on the top line of the paper, it wasn't likely to be the first time the child had ever written it.

If, indeed, it was the child who had been practicing.

And as Carol held her memory of that piece of paper, another of her senses suddenly came into play.

Touch.

She could recall the *feel* of the paper, smooth and supple. Not rough and brittle. *New* paper, she realized with a start, not old enough for a woman who had died at twenty-two to have used when she was six or seven. . . .

Carol's eyes darted over the lines of photographs, looking for one identical to the picture she had seen in the frame at Miller's house. The *only* photograph she had seen there . . .

A suspicion too vague to articulate was suddenly percolating in her mind. But it was driven from consciousness when she found, in the middle of the bottom row of victims, the matching picture, the pretty brown-haired girl. At the bottom edge of the portrait a label was pasted with the name typed on it. And there it was: Suzanne-with-a-z.

It took just another moment before the woman's last name registered. *Hollister.* The name on the label wasn't Miller . . . but Suzanne Hollister.

Carol stared at the image of the young woman superimposed in memory with its twin, on the dresser in the room where she had slept—and where she had let Paul Miller make love to her. A wave of nausea rose through her, as if she had been tossed and pitched for too long on a wild and perilous voyage.

Carol spun away. Perhaps the explanation was a simple one, nothing sinister. A married name! Miller hadn't mentioned that his daughter was married . . . but the one time they had talked about it, he hadn't been concerned with any details, only his daughter's bright future—a medical student, hadn't he said?—a future that had been brutally cut short.

Yet that childish handwriting had been scribbled across a piece of paper that was not aged and yellowed. . . .

Carol scanned the table on the other side of the room. Folders hung on wire racks, files relating to the victims. She hesitated barely a second before bolting across the floor and putting her hands to the file that was tabbed "Hollister."

She could imagine one reason after another to explain Paul Miller's behavior from the day he had first appeared before her and asked her to inscribe a book to Suzanne-with-a-z. But none of the reasons she gave herself could possibly be good enough.

29

"LOOK FOR A PLACE where the river is miles wide," the man had told her on the phone, "and there are big cliffs visible on the other side."

This was the first time the Hudson River had broken into view since Carol had left New York almost an hour ago, and from the broad vista she knew it must be the place she had been told to expect. She drove on only another minute until, on a side road off the highway, she spotted the next landmark—a large sign reading CROTON COLONIAL DINER. A quarter mile beyond, she veered onto the exit ramp.

The diner was a low building with a flat roof rimmed by a white wooden border, and two wings extending from either side of the stepped-up central entrance. To one side was a large parking lot. Only when Carol turned into the lot and saw that almost every place was taken did she realize it must be the lunch hour.

She had no appetite herself, had lost all sense of time since Paul Miller had brought her back to the city. After discovering that the girl Miller claimed as his daughter did not share his name, there had been nothing on her mind but to learn why. Snooping in the files, she had discovered that Suzanne Hollister had been—as Miller had claimed—a medical student at the University of Connecticut at the time of her abduction. A note stapled to an autopsy form indicated that personal effects belonging to the victim, currently held as evidence, were registered as the property of her husband, Kenneth Hollister.

Surreptitiously, Carol had made a note of the address and phone number given for the husband. She had meant to race straight out of the offices of the task force, but then Eric had reappeared. Paul Miller, he told her, had not turned up at the New Jersey state police with Frank Matheson's travel logs. This, added to Carol's other concerns, left her more disoriented than ever. Why would Paul withhold evidence that would help Tommy?

All the time she was making her statement—about what she had seen in Frank Matheson's trunk, and Margot's mention of planning a foray into Frank's home—Carol couldn't stop thinking about whether to share with Eric her new questions about Miller. In the end she had kept them to herself. To say anything, she feared, might lead Eric to conclude that she and Miller had spent the night together, and whatever the cost to her own comfort or safety, hurting Eric was the last thing in the world she would willingly do. If anything good had come out of this nightmare, it had been meeting him.

After completing her statement, she told Eric that she was due in Long Island to take care of her father's transfer to a nursing home. From the lobby of the federal office building, however, she had called the telephone number given for Suzanne Hollister's husband—a number with a 914 area code, which included the Westchester and Duchess county suburbs. The call had brought her to the diner.

By a cashier's desk just inside the entrance, a burly man in tinted glasses stopped Carol and asked in heavily accented English if she wanted to sit in a booth or at the counter.

"I'm looking for Ken Hollister," Carol said.

"I tell him," the man replied. "Wait at counter."

She took a stool and ordered coffee from a waitress.

The cup had no sooner been set in front of her than a slight blond man dressed in chinos and a white tennis shirt emerged from the kitchen accompanied by the cashier. As he came over alone, Carol thought how young he looked to have already lost a wife.

"Miss Warren, I'm Ken Hollister." He offered his hand and Carol took it. "I hope you didn't mind meeting here." On the phone he had explained that he worked afternoons at the diner as assistant manager, helping to pay his tuition for graduate courses in geology.

"Not at all," Carol said.

"I won't be able to give you much time. This is our busiest hour."

"I won't need long, Mr. Hollister." Carol hesitated. On the phone she had been too timid to reveal her true reason for wanting to see him. So she had misled him, saying she was "calling from the task force," and that she needed to interview him to "fill in a couple of blanks" in their background on the victim.

Sitting down, Ken Hollister filled the pause. "I've spoken to your people so many times in the last couple of years, Miss Warren, I'm amazed there's still any ground left to cover."

The lie should have come easily enough—always some stone unturned, couldn't be too thorough in an investigation like this. But Carol couldn't bring herself to go on deceiving him.

"Mr. Hollister," she said after a second. "I'm not really with the task force. I need the information for myself."

"Yourself?" A wince tightened his face. "What are you—a reporter? Looking for some gruesome new angle to give your readers a few thrills?" He was half off the stool already.

"Please don't go." She grabbed his arm. "I just need to know a couple of things."

"I'm sick of you reporters," he said angrily. "If this

isn't going to help catch the guy who killed Suze, then I don't give a shit." He shook his head. "You people don't seem to get it. The pain never stops, not for any of us who loved her. But you exploit that, don't you, because you know the only thing that makes it bearable is to think that somehow we can help—"

"Please believe me, Mr. Hollister," Carol said, "I'm not a reporter and I do understand your pain. I really do."

Her voice must have conveyed heartfelt comprehension, for Hollister settled back onto the stool. "What's this about?"

"Catching your wife's killer," Carol said. "I want to see that done every bit as much as you do. I swear it. My best friend was also a victim."

He gave her a searching look, then glanced over his shoulder as if making sure that business would tolerate his absence. "Okay," he said. "A few questions."

Carol was relieved that he had not pressed for more details about her motives. To admit she was the sister of a suspect might alienate him again.

"You mentioned other people who cared about your wife," she said. "I wonder who you were referring to."

He gave her another curious glance. "Well . . . the rest of her family, of course."

"Her three brothers?"

"Yeah. They took it very hard—kid sister and all."

So that much was true, Carol was glad to hear. "And their father? What was his reaction?"

"Thank God, he never had to deal with it."

"Never . . . ?"

"He died when Suze was seventeen."

Carol gazed at the young man blankly, her head crowded all at once with so many thoughts that she couldn't form words. The old edition of *Mother Goose* with the child's name scrawled in front. The picture on the dresser at Miller's house.

And that bedroom . . .

As if her mind were taking her back, leading her into that room, she rotated on the stool and turned through the imaginary door, and she was there again seeing the charming decor, smelling the freshly washed towels. Her arm floated out as though to pick up the framed photograph again—and knocked with a loud clatter against the coffee cup on the counter. She became aware of Hollister looking at her with puzzled concern.

"Her name," Carol said abruptly. "Your wife's maiden name. What was it?"

"Conroy."

"Suzanne Conroy," Carol echoed.

Hollister nodded.

Carol looked down and shook her head. When the silence had lasted several seconds, Hollister said, "I have to get back to work. Before I go, do you want to tell me what this is all about?"

"I wish I could," she said very quietly. "I wish to God I knew."

She was barely aware of his rising from his stool and moving away.

Absently she blotted with a napkin at her spilled coffee, still dwelling on the room where she had spent last night. Like a movie set, she reflected, a closed-off area of make-believe constructed to sustain a false drama. Yet that scene was only the last act of the story. And it couldn't have worked if other scenes hadn't been played first. . . .

Lumley. The bookseller who had described Miller's coming into his shop, buying books for his children—three boys and a girl. Why had George Lumley abetted the lie, told her that Suzanne was Paul Miller's daughter?

After paying her check, Carol asked the cashier if there was a public telephone. He pointed to an alcove in a corner by the rest rooms. Carol exchanged two dollars for quarters and went to the phone.

"I don't know any Mr. Lumley," said the young salesman at the Wordsong bookstore who answered her call. "But would you like to speak to the owner's wife, Mrs. Carswell?"

The owner's wife? Carswell? "Yes, I would," Carol said, trying to sound matter-of-fact.

The woman who came on the line was the same one who had answered the first time and taken a message for George Lumley. Carol spoke briskly, even trying to sound tough. "Mrs. Carswell, this is Carol Warren. I'm trying to reach George Lumley. When I called two weeks ago, you took a message."

"Yes," she said, "and George isn't in today. I'll tell him you tried to reach him again."

"But I called you because these are business hours, Mrs. Carswell, and I believed that the owner of the store might be there. That was before your salesman told me that the *real* owner is your husband."

There was a pause. "We're partners," the woman said unsteadily. "My husband and Mr. Lumley. Now, Miss Warren, if you need to talk to George, I'll tell him you called." She hung up.

Partners? Or was that only a last futile try at improvisation? From the woman's abrupt manner it was clear that she was embarrassed at being confronted.

As Carol left the diner, the questions tumbled through her brain. Why had the owners of a bookstore been willing to aid Paul Miller's deception? Why, even before that, had Miller wanted to pass off Suzanne Hollister as his daughter? To explain his single-minded devotion to tracking down a serial murderer? Now, like every other thing Miller had ever told her, she knew it wasn't true. No child of his had suffered at the hands of the Deep Woods Killer.

So what kept Miller going, what fueled an obsession

that was no less mad in its way than the killer's bloodlust?

Carol got into her car, drove south toward her father's house. Coming out of the shifting confusions of the day, the journey toward absolute sadness almost seemed a relief.

Arms drooping limply at his sides, he was waiting on the living room couch when she arrived. His tan anorak lay across his knees, and his good winter gloves were placed beside him so he wouldn't forget them. On the floor, one to each side, were his old Samsonite suitcases.

To be torn from his moorings was so cruel, she thought. Why couldn't he finish out his years in this house?

She bent to kiss him. "Hi, Daddy, I'm sorry I'm late."

"Are you?" Pete asked, looking up at her. "What time is it?" He lifted his retirement Rolex to his face. Gazing at it, he tilted his head to one side, then the other. "No, you're not late," he said.

He had no idea what time it was, Carol realized, but despite his weakness he still clung to his pride.

She sat and put her arm around him, and he rested his head on her shoulder. This was surely one of the worst moments of her life. "Tommy couldn't make it today," she said with forced good cheer, "but he'll come see you next week."

"Tommy," Pete Warren said simply, as though needing a moment to register the name. "Fine boy. He must be busy with his work."

There could be no solace in her father's illness, Carol realized, but she discovered one saving grace: At least he had remained ignorant of Tommy's troubles.

Mrs. Briggs descended the stairs, dressed up for her last day with Pete Warren. Her stocky frame was draped in a plain gray dress and a gold necklace instead of the usual T-shirt and slacks. "Hello, Miss Warren," she said.

"Hi, Mrs. Briggs." Carol stood. "You're looking lovely today."

"Thank you, I wanted Pete to have a nice send-off."

"It's very thoughtful of you," Carol replied. "I guess everything's . . . ready."

"Yes," Mrs. Briggs said plainly, compassion evident in her sorrowful face, "it's all in order. I'll just wait in the back until . . ."

"I think we'll have one last look around," Carol said. "How about it, Daddy?"

Pete didn't answer immediately. He reached over to the larger of the two suitcases and flipped the worn handle back and forth. "Let's do that," he said suddenly, putting his jacket aside and standing up.

As he moved through his own bedroom, through Carol's and Tommy's rooms, he touched an object here and there—Tommy's baseball pennants, Carol's child-sized drawing board. In the hallway he stopped at the wall of bookshelves.

"Built these myself," he said, "with lumber from Uncle Culley's store."

Pete ran his finger along the spines of the books. When he touched the editions of the Dana stories, Carol had a faint echo of seeing her books on another shelf—no, not a shelf, a table, the end table in George Lumley's house. She remembered autographing them, the old copy of *Tiger, Tiger* and the newer ones from Lumley's store.

Why, Carol wondered now, would he have brought them from there? If, as Lumley said, he and his wife had been admiring and collecting Carol's work for a long time, why was only one of the books old and all the rest new? That, too, made no sense, unless George Lumley had never collected her books at all.

Pete was starting downstairs. Carol trailed him into

the small study off the kitchen, then back, retracing his steps, into the dining room. He picked up a silver-framed photograph from the sideboard—Carol and Tommy as children, hanging on to their mother's arms.

"You kids," Pete said, "I couldn't have asked for better . . . a daughter and a son. It never mattered to me, I never regretted it."

He set the picture down, his hand resting on the frame.

Carol turned to him. "Never regretted what, Daddy?" she asked. "What never mattered?"

"I loved your mother, and that was that," Pete replied, oblivious to Carol. "Not a love everyone could understand, but you can't say it didn't work. It worked for us."

"Daddy, of course it did."

Pete stared at the picture for one long moment, then took his hand away and strode into the living room. "Carrie, the sun's starting to go down, didn't you say we were late?" He looked at his suitcases. "Where are we going?" he asked.

At the nursing home Carol helped her father unpack his clothes into the small dresser that had been brought from the house, then led him out for a walk on the back lawn. Dusk was settling, but the asphalt paths were lighted by enclosed bulbs close to the ground.

"Too bad Tommy couldn't be here today," Pete said.

"Daddy, he wanted to be—"

"You two used to play right over there," Pete said, pointing to a patch of trees. "And he climbed that rope to you. You kids had a lot of fun in this yard."

Carol felt the sting in the corner of her eyes. Pete was still at home, and to him this lawn was the back-yard.

"Tommy was crackerjack," he said, "just cracker-jack. I never had a single regret."

Again the mention of regret. "About what, Daddy?"

Her father went on scanning the trees. "Living here," he said, turning to Carol with a serious look, "this had to be best the way to work things out, isn't that right?"

Now he meant the nursing home, she thought. He had accepted it. "Yes," she said, "it's for the best."

"For all of us," Pete Warren went on, "not just the kid, good for her and me. Good for Culley, too."

No, this was something else. The kid. Did her father mean Tommy? And how did Culley Nelson come into it?

But when she asked, her father turned back to the main building of the nursing home and said maybe Culley would visit him here. "I'm hungry," Pete announced abruptly. "What time do they serve dinner?"

She stayed until just past eight o'clock, when one of the nurses suggested that she ought to leave and allow Pete to get settled in. At the front door she said good-bye. Hugging her, Pete promised to drive into the city, see a show with her, unaware that he had no car, had not driven himself in almost two years.

On the sidewalk Carol waved to him, and he smiled and waved back, then disappeared into the building. It was now that Carol accepted the truth. Her father was descending into an ever darkening fog; bringing him here had indeed been the best thing. No matter how unpleasant facts were, sometimes they had to be faced.

IN THE DEEP WOODS

Can you see me now, my love?

He looked into the wide green eyes as he lifted her head slowly by the tendrils of long brown hair woven through his fingers, lifted it until the mouth was next to his, and he kissed the lips very lightly, upper then lower since the mouth was open wide. They were still warm, pliant, though the pink circle was held taut with a scream. As it had been at the moment when the nerves gave their final command.

He moved the head away, dangled it at arm's length as an ancient sentry on a battlement might hoist a lantern in the dark, and he stared for a longer time into the eyes.

It fascinated him always. At what moment did they cease to see? Never, he believed at moments like this. Never. She always saw.

She saw him now. If she loved him, she would always see him—keep an eye on him, that was what she used to say as he ran up the street, if he remembered correctly. When she died, they had closed her eyes. But he wanted them open. As they were now.

So let me show you how I love you. . . .

He lowered the head and used the open mouth as he always did, and when he was finished he put it down so the eyes were looking up through the thick lacework of branches to the sky.

It was over. The act complete. She had seen how much he loved her, the sacrifice he was willing to make, chances to take. Shown her how smart he could be, too. And of course, how perfectly charming. He couldn't have done it without charm.

He started to circle the small open area under the trees, collecting his possessions, scouring for stray clues, cleaning up.

He chuckled softly as he heard her again in memory, murmuring that favorite homily—always when she would wrap him in a towel after a bath, warm him with an embrace, and rub him dry. Oh yes, darling, cleanliness is next to godliness. Around and around the little clearing he went, and as he walked, he hummed the old song that always came to mind at this stage, her voice crooning the lyric once more.

I'm in the mood for love . . .

Time and again he scuffed over the ground, bent over to peer more closely at every place he had stood, had set anything down. Even after there was nothing more to see than bloodied leaves and stones—nothing more except the corpse and the head—he kept circling. Always be clean.

Simply because you're near me . . .

Perfect, he mused proudly, as he backed up at last to the edge of the clearing for his final inspection.

Turning his back on what he had done, he began making his way back to where he had left the car.

And suddenly the realization came. He didn't have the feeling today, no sense of completion and satisfaction, release and resolution.

He wanted her to watch him again. Needed it right now.

30 THE PHONE WAS RINGING when Carol came into her apartment. She sat down on the bed and simply listened to it ring and ring. For some reason she felt certain the caller was Paul Miller, wanting to apologize again, or declare his love for her, or maybe tell her that he had more evidence against Frank. And she knew that the sound of his voice would crack her apart, that of all her confusions the deepest sprang from last night, when she had trusted him enough to accept him into her arms.

Hadn't all those women trusted someone, too, the man with the gift of charm? Wasn't that how he lured them—before he killed them?

Dear God, with her own tragedies—with Dad and Margot and Tommy—wasn't there some way to cleanse these killings from her thoughts?

She forced herself to look for the light, to concentrate on brighter moments. *No regrets*, her father had said.

And what had he called Tommy? *Just crackerjack* . . .

Impelled by the reminder of her father's memories, Carol rose from the bed and drifted across the room to her closet. On her tiptoes, she reached up and felt across the top shelf until her hand touched the old shoebox where she kept her own collection of family snapshots. She pulled it down and carried it to the living room. Sitting by the terrace door, she upended the box and began to sift through the old pictures, just like the ones in Pete Warren's album.

Here she was, standing in the backyard with Tommy. How old were they—seven and eight? Now she came to Uncle Culley at Coney Island, standing in front of the Ferris wheel with Tommy on his shoulders. Then a wedding pose of Mom and Dad, champagne glasses held high.

. . . not a love everyone could understand, her father had said.

Listening to her father's voice, she realized that the nightmare was still with her. She wasn't looking at the pictures for relief or distraction. She was looking for clues.

. . . not just the kid, good for her . . . and Culley, too . . .

But what clues? What connections was she making?

She piled the old pictures into the box. Then, as if obliterating the past could cleanse it of all mysteries, she violently thrust the box away, sending it flying, scattering photographs across the floor.

The clanging chime fell into her sleep like a bomb detonating over a sleeping city.

The front door.

Drowsily Carol swung her legs over the edge of the bed, stretched to get her robe. The glowing green numbers on the digital clock said 2:24.

She was in the foyer, reaching to remove the safety chain on the door, when her mental alarm went off and she came fully awake. Who could be ringing her bell at this hour? How had they gotten past the doorman? She left the chain in place as she turned the deadbolt.

"Who is it?" she called out as she opened the door a crack and peered into the hall. In her hazy focus the first thing she saw was the bulky overcoat, then the grey homburg.

"Go away," Carol shouted hoarsely. "I don't want you here, I don't want you near me."

She tried to close the door, but Miller was pushing against it.

"Carol, wait!"

She leaned harder, pressing with the full weight of her body, but the door wouldn't budge. Taking a step away, she slammed her shoulder against the metal panel. It shut. Before she could throw the deadbolt, Miller was trying to turn the knob, but it was latched and didn't move.

"Carol, it's essential that I speak with you. I tried to reach you today."

"Leave me alone!" she shouted through the door. "You liar, you goddamned liar—"

"Please, Carol, whatever has changed your mind about me, I can explain if you'll give me a chance. Listen to me, there's been more killing. Last night . . ."

Last night. When they had been together.

Carol leaned against the closed door for another moment. Then she undid the locks and opened it, though she left the safety chain in place.

Paul went on, laying his hand against the doorframe and talking through the narrow opening. "A young woman disappeared from a shopping mall north of Philadelphia," he said. "An hour later, at another mall farther north, a second woman was reported missing. It's happening, Carol—the frenzy. The bodies were found this morning. A utility crew repairing a damaged line, they found both of them in a gully off the highway. The killer tried to do a quick burial, but it didn't work."

Carol simply stared at him. Did she dare believe anything he said?

"I've checked with the phone company, Carol, and you called your brother this morning. He's not at home and I need to find him. Where did he go?"

"I don't know anything!" she cried. "I never did. But it's Frank! My brother is innocent."

Miller shoved hard at the door, as though forgetting it was held by the chain. "Carol, goddamnit, you have to help me. The killer is starting to feel cornered now, and more women are going to die unless you tell me where he is. You know, don't you—you know where Tommy has gone? You've got to help me find him!"

There was no reason to trust Miller. "Who are you to be making accusations?" she shouted. "You're not Suzanne Hollister's father. Her husband never heard of you."

"I'll explain all that," Miller replied urgently, "but not now. Nothing matters but finding your brother before—"

"Why?" Carol demanded, her voice raw. "What about Frank, the evidence—"

Miller cut her off. "Those travel records, Carol, they were dummied up . . . changed. I talked to the police and saw Frank Matheson myself. I checked his own records, his gasoline credit card receipts. It was your brother, Carol, he fixed those logs to shift suspicion to Matheson."

"What about the bloodstains in Frank's trunk?" Carol demanded. "And the cane? And that psychiatrist? Tommy took a test, it proved he isn't a killer."

Miller slipped his hand through the door, wrapping his fingers around the edge. "There are answers for everything, Carol, if you'll just let me explain."

"No!" she screamed.

He gave her a measuring glance. "Carol, after last night . . ."

"You rotten bastard, don't you ever talk to me about what happened last night—making love to me in that room, playing on my sympathy with that goddamn phony room and that phony picture. I don't know why you're doing this to me, but you're crazy, Paul. Go away."

Slowly he yielded, slid his hand away from the frame and pulled the door shut.

Imagining that he might still be waiting outside, might hurl his bulk at the door and burst in, Carol went on standing in the foyer for a long time.

*　　*　　*

The family photographs and mementos dotted the living room rug. Stepping between them to the terrace doors, she picked up the phone and carried it to the couch. Three o'clock in the morning, she thought, they'll all be asleep.

But she turned the looseleaf pages of her leatherbound directory, found the number, and made the call to Vermont.

It rang a long time at the other end, then was answered in a groggy rasp. "Hello . . ."

"Jill, is that you? It's Carol."

"Carol . . . my God, it's the middle of the night."

"I know. I'm sorry. But . . . I needed to talk to Tommy, to know he's all right."

"He left hours ago," Jill replied flatly. "He said he had to meet you tomorrow to close the sale of your father's house."

"Did you talk, work anything out?"

"Carol, there is nothing—"

"But with the baby coming! Jill, this whole thing is—"

"Don't, Carol. There's no point in hoping I'll change my mind. I don't want to have him near me ever again. It's over."

Carol's eyes had been roaming over the pictures scattered on the floor. Near her feet lay several of Jill and Tommy in happier days. As she spoke, Carol's gaze rested on one showing them in bathing suits, sunning themselves in the backyard of the house on Lloyd's Neck Road.

"He's going to be cleared of all this, Jill. Maybe soon. Will you give him a chance then?"

"Carol, I know who he is now. I see him for what he is. I don't want to talk to you anymore about it, so I'm hanging up. And please don't call me again." There was a brief pause. "Ever," she added right before Carol heard the click.

*   *   *

Through the terrace doors the strong autumn wind blew, swirling gusts of the cold that afflicted the city in the hours before dawn. It came blowing in off the Atlantic Ocean, coiled up the Hudson River, and swept across the concrete grid of the city, magnified in force as it funneled through the canyons of tall buildings.

Carol stood by the open doors, watching the lights blinking through the darkness, feeling the wind rush over her face and arms. If only it could fully wake her, she thought, rouse her to some higher level of mental acuity where she would finally see the answer clear to saving her brother.

On the edge of her drawing table pictures of Dana were piled, and the air gusting through the door snatched them up and lifted them, sending them floating across the room. Mingled with the old photographs, they troubled her mind, caused her to sift through the past, decisions made, decisions avoided, men she had loved and never married, men she had spurned and who had spurned her. The images of the pictures that had been born in her mind, and those that had been born out of living, kept spinning past her eyes, a blizzard in her brain, even after the papers from the drawing table had settled to the floor.

And then, as if it were a single crystalline snowflake that had landed and stuck on a flat surface, one moment was frozen in her mind's eye, with all the lines and shadows of its design sharply defined. . . .

Her mother, cradling Tommy in her arms, crooning a sweet song to him. Carol could almost hear the melody, too. Not the usual children's lullaby. Something almost . . . seductive.

Now the feelings flooded back. The little girl she had been was standing by her mother's side, wanting to be cradled like that, yearning to have a song sung to her, for her. Oh, Mommy, a small voice in Carol cried to the present that was past, to the sweet singer who was forever silent.

Forget it, Carol told herself. No use, she said unspoken. She was aware of how unusual it was to experience those past feelings—and of how she experienced them in ways that held them at bay. For suddenly she understood as never before that the little girl she had grown up to become, little Dana, had spent years fighting her way through forests and underground caves, across oceans, through worlds hidden beneath the surface of the earth, always searching for what she had missed herself: the source of protection and perfect love. Her mother, who had died leaving her alone.

Yet why, when she looked back on it, did it seem that Tommy hadn't been abandoned as she had? Only because the song had been sung to him?

The wind was making her shiver now. The wind— and somehow, too, the memory of the music. In a quick, almost violent move Carol pulled the terrace door shut, blocking the wind.

31 A VOICE SQUAWKED LOUDLY across the lumberyard through speakers attached to the side of the warehouse. "Culley Nelson, visitor at the front office."

An engine backfired somewhere nearby, and Carol turned to see a flatbed truck piled with window frames pulling away from the loading dock. Her eyes scanned across the other activity in the yard, forklifts moving back and forth taking lumber and siding from stacks of material arrayed around her. People were building houses, Carol thought, putting things together, enlarging their lives—while her life was crumbling.

When she had phoned him this morning at his lumberyard in Long Island City, Culley had dodged her questions.

"Carol, honey, why are you so fired up about this so early on a nice sunny morning?" Pete Warren's ramblings, Culley had insisted, could only be attributed to his disease.

But in Culley's evasions and pleas of ignorance, Carol heard a telltale hesitation. Something lay hidden in the spaces between his words, she believed, a truth she needed urgently to hear.

He came across the yard toward her with his big head down, a cigarette dangling from the corner of his mouth. The driver of the flatbed truck intervened, holding out a clipboard while Culley slipped off his heavy yellow workgloves and scrawled a signature.

Continuing on toward Carol, he tossed his cigarette

onto the cinder-covered ground and crushed it with his heel.

"Carol, sweetie, whyn't you tell me you're coming? When we spoke a couple hours ago—"

"I didn't buy it, Culley," Carol said with quiet force. "That's why I'm here. You're hiding something, I could tell when we talked on the phone. You thought I could be put off. But I can't. I need answers, I really need them badly."

Culley glanced away to the piles of timber stacked around him, then his eyes came back and held Carol's for a long, silent moment. He shook his head slightly—not a refusal, Carol thought, but almost an expression of sympathy, the sort of gesture one made unconsciously when passing a bad traffic accident. "Let's go inside," he murmured at last.

He led her past cartons piled high on wooden skids, around the perimeter of the warehouse to the back. Here, away from the noise of the yard, was a small office—a desk covered with order forms and empty soda cans, two scuffed bankers' chairs on casters, and on a junk table in a corner a Burns coffee maker with a glass pot of steaming water.

"Want some hot chocolate?" Culley asked as he shed his brown duffel coat and hung it on a wall hook. "Nothing like hot chocolate on a day like this."

Making conversation, Carol felt, delaying.

"That'd be great, Culley," she said, sitting down.

"Looks like you could really use it," he observed as he went to the pot in the corner.

"I didn't sleep much last night. Or the night before."

He gave her a worried look, yet said nothing. It was so unlike Culley—not to ask exactly what was causing her sleeplessness—that her last shadow of doubt was purged. There was some guilty secret that had lain hidden for years.

Culley busied himself opening packets of powder,

making hot chocolate in two chipped white mugs. Killing more time, Carol mused. But she waited patiently.

Finally he passed her a mug and a napkin and took the chair opposite her, rolling it backward to the wall. He dipped his head to take a sip of the hot chocolate. "So," he said without looking up.

"So," Carol said. "What did Dad mean yesterday? All this talk of 'no regrets.' It wasn't just his mind playing tricks, was it?"

Culley set his mug on the desk, dug into his shirt pocket for his ever-present pack of Camels, and shook one into his palm.

"Sweetie," he said then, "why is this all of a sudden the biggest thing on your mind?"

"It's not the biggest thing," Carol replied. "It's just part of a lot of things I'm trying to figure out." She raised the pitch of intensity in her voice. "Culley, Dad said something about how everything had worked out for the best, staying here, how it worked out for you, too. As if there'd once been a choice—even a need— to go somewhere else. Why would that be, Culley? What worked out by staying?"

He leaned sideways, slid his hand into the pocket of his pants, and retrieved his Zippo lighter. He flipped it open, lit the cigarette, inhaled deeply, and leaned far forward, blowing the smoke down at the floor.

Carol pulled herself to the edge of her chair. "Culley, I need the truth. Whatever you've been keeping from me—you and Dad—I've got to have it now. I'm mixed up about a lot of things, and this is important if I'm going to see things clear—"

He raised his eyes as he rode over her plea. "Carol, it's all done now, finished. There's no percentage in dredging anything up."

On the brink of insisting, she considered dropping it as Culley suggested. Turn the clock back, forget what her father had said. Yet the perceptions of last night kept Carol rooted to the chair. She could run from this—but she had been running all her life, running through a dark forest where unseen evil things lurked around her. Today she wanted finally to see into the forest, to stop fleeing from the unknown.

"I have to decide for myself," she said, "what the percentage is. Tell me what Dad meant, Culley, so I can make that decision."

He smiled ruefully. "You know, hon, I always figured you for a softie. But you're givin' me one helluva surprise right now. You're no softie, are ya?"

"I used to be," she said calmly. "But then, I used to believe that all things and people were pretty much what they seemed—that the only monsters in the world were the ones I made up. That's not the way it is, though, Culley . . . is it?"

He took another drag on his cigarette, then dropped the butt into an old Coke can on the desk. "No, baby, some things ain't what they seem." He stood, pushed his chair away, and turned toward the wall. "Oh boy," he said. He covered his face with his hands and rubbed his cheeks as if he were trying to grate the skin away. "Oh boy. Was I ever hopin' to go to my grave and never talk about none of this."

He turned around and leaned against the wall. "I made a mistake, kid, a bad mistake. A lifetime ago, thirty-five years. I was a happily married man, and I had two kids, and I did a dumb thing. I had an affair with . . . with Jeanne Simpson."

Carol heard the name as if called out to her from the end of a long tunnel. "My mother? You had an affair with my mother?"

"She wasn't your mom then. She was just the prettiest girl in town."

"But thirty-five years ago," Carol said slowly, "Mom and Dad were married."

"Not yet, not that winter. Jeanne and Pete were dating, he was pretty far gone on her and he'd already

proposed, but they weren't married yet." Culley lit another cigarette, and for a moment his eyes clouded
over, as if he were looking back into time. "I don't
know what we thought we were doing, how she and
I hooked up while she was seeing your dad. It had no
place to go, we both knew that. But she got pregnant,
Carol. And what could I do? Get a divorce? I already
had the two boys, it would have ruined everybody's
life. In those days you couldn't go around the corner
and get an abortion, not like now . . . and anyway, your
mom didn't want one. She figured maybe she could—
well, give Pete a chance to believe the kid was his. But
there wasn't enough time for that, so she told him the
truth. You can think bad of your mom when you hear
this, but it was a brave thing, telling Pete. And he married her, knowing about it . . . because he loved her,
he really did." Culley's voice thickened a little as he
went on. "Tell you the truth, Carol, he loved her better than I did. And the both of 'em, they cared for you
and Tommy just the same, you have to know that,
nothin' ever affected the way they loved you kids."

Carol felt lost, adrift. She was floating out to sea,
alone on a raft, and there was no anchor, nothing to
grab hold of.

Culley, the family's dear friend . . . Tommy's real
father.

And her own father had let Culley play the role of
uncle, of benefactor. They had taken vacations together, given parties for each other. My God, Uncle
Culley had been best man at their wedding. What had
these people been doing, what kind of lives had they
been living?

"Culley," she said, "I can't . . . it's so hard to absorb
this."

Culley sat down and rolled his chair close. "Sweetie,
you wanted to know. But your folks and I, we always
thought it would be better to keep it buried. Maybe
that was wrong. But now you're gettin' the lesson. A

lot of what you kids think life is, it's just grown-ups pretending. We tell you things are gonna be fine, and we try to make 'em look that way . . . and then you learn. It's just the way life is. We made mistakes, and we tried to fix 'em the only way we could. We did our best." He put out his hands, palms upward, a gesture that expressed an odd indifference. "That's all."

Carol was searching her memory for any sign she might have been given, any inkling of a message from her parents. But as always, she recalled her childhood only in fragments, isolated flashes of light. No, she had never known. But who was this mother she had loved so dearly—this woman in love with one man, willing to marry him, who had already slept with another, conceived his child?

Had Tommy sensed it? With all of Culley's attention . . .

"Do you think Tommy knows?" she asked.

"No way. Your folks and I, we made a pact, the three of us, to keep the secret, never to tell. Your dad's sick now, Carol, but he's no fool, no way he was gonna tell Tom." Culley grabbed her hands, held them. "And don't you be the one to tell him, sweetie, there's no good purpose to it. It was best then to leave everybody in the dark, wasn't it? And it shoulda stayed that way. It worked out for everybody in the end, Carol, it worked out for all of us, a lot of lives saved that might've been destroyed."

Carol stood up, put her mug on the desk. "Thank you, Culley. I'm glad you could tell me."

He got up, held himself away for another moment, then took her in an embrace. "Thank *you,* sweetie. If it was me in your shoes, I don't know as I'd be takin' this the way you are. I worried about how you kids would grow up, and now I know you turned out all right."

*   *   *

Walking to her car, Carol wondered what effect those secrets could have had on Tommy . . . on her. A father pretending, another father competing, a mother with her love child. As Carol reached the parking lot, she looked back and saw that Culley was outside the warehouse, watching her. Again she heard his last words: *a pact to keep the secret . . . a lot of lives saved.*

But how many lives, she couldn't help thinking as she waved good-bye, had this secret finally cost?

32 TAKING THE TURN into the long drive of Tommy's house, Carol saw that the mailbox near the main road bulged with magazines and advertising fliers. On the way to Saddle River she had stopped twice to telephone. Each time the phone had gone unanswered—though there had been plenty of time for Tommy to drive back from Vermont. Some black intuition warned that his absence might be due to a fatal accident on the road. Only it wasn't an accident that worried her so much as a catastrophe of another kind. She gunned her car up the drive.

For all the newness of the big modern house, a forlorn atmosphere already hovered over it. Drifts of moldy leaves lay clotted in the parking circle fronting the entrance, and newspapers had mounted on the threshold, faded and swollen from moisture. Using the key Tommy had given her at his housewarming, Carol let herself in. Even knowing the house was empty, she was moved by an accustomed respect for privacy to give a ritual call from the high-ceilinged entrance hall.

"Tommy . . . hello? Anyone home?" Her voice traveled away to the far reaches of the house.

She glanced around, took in the small brushstrokes of a life interrupted—a scarf thrown over the banister, a shopping bag in the kitchen doorway full of empty soda bottles to be returned for deposit. And as she heard the echoes of her footsteps on the parquet floor, another chilling premonition came to her. This house would never be lived in again, not by anyone she knew. Jill was gone, never coming back. Nor was Tommy.

Carol shivered as though feeling the touch of a ghost on her shoulder, a spirit that nudged her forward. She started to climb the stairs and was halfway up when she understood where she was going and why. Prowling. Questing. Looking for truth in the inanimate shell of a man's life, the shape it took around him in the place where he found refuge. If this man— not wholly her brother, she reminded herself, yet surely still her blood—if he could be the elusive monster so many were seeking, wouldn't this place show some sign of it, some clinging spoor of an animal hidden in a corner of his lair?

She went from room to room, opening closets and drawers and cabinets, sweeping her eyes over every surface.

There was nothing out of the ordinary. Closets filled with his clothes and Jill's, drawers littered with innocuous mail, stray snapshots of a man and his wife on a vacation in Mexico, and standing in the skeletal frame of the house during construction. Carol moved from one room to the next—some furnished, some not—bedrooms for children who would never be born, guests who would never come.

Or would they? Having searched through the second floor, Carol felt her mood lift. What began as premonitions might be nothing more than gloomy fantasies. Here, in these private spaces, all was normal, so absolutely banal. All as it would be in any house where the owners were absent, the routine ruptured. Perhaps there was hope for repair? Did the discovery of a secret kept by one generation have to mean that shame and evil lay waiting to be exposed in another?

She went to the landing, about to descend again, then glanced at the narrow half-flight of stairs that led to the attic. The space under the roof wasn't finished, she remembered Tommy saying, but he'd planned a little hideaway up there—or when there were kids, maybe a rec room with a Ping-Pong table. As if she only wanted to see what had been done with the space rather than hunt for markers of guilt, Carol started up.

The area was still unfinished, the pads of insulation stapled between the canted roofbeams not yet covered. But someone was using the space for a study. Next to the row of dormer windows running along one side, a rectangular table had been placed, a dark oak piece of bric-a-brac. On the tabletop stood an uneven stack of books, a gooseneck lamp with a red-enameled metal shade, and a cup of pencils. A spiral notebook lay open at the center, in front of a chair facing the door. On one of the pages several lists had been scrawled.

Carol walked over to the table, turned the notebook around, and read the rows of penciled words written in clear, flowing script. Tommy's handwriting, she thought.

Woman looking out window, man staring at her was on the top line. Carol picked up the book, her eyes scanning the lines below:

Two children playing in yard
Woman in hat at ticket window
Man with stick in hand and jumping dog

One after another, the bizarre descriptive phrases marched down to the bottom of the page.

Fireman climbing ladder
Man and woman wading
Child curled on a bed

Beside each, at the border, was a small checkmark.

Her wall against comprehension stood intact for one more moment, then cracked. Slowly Carol's gaze wandered from the page to the stack of books. She noted slips of yellow paper sticking out, marking places in each one, as she began reading the titles on the spines: *Behavioral Psychology, Adolescent Psychiatry,*

Diagnostic Testing, Case Histories in Sociopathology. Carol
tossed the notebook down and snatched up the book
on top of the stack. Knocking the cover back to expose
the flyleaf, she saw "Return to Jill Warren" written inside. For just a second the tightness across her chest
eased as she revised her perceptions. *Jill's* books. This
was *her* place to study.

But it was too late to repair the crack in the wall
against knowledge and reason. Even before Carol
picked up the volume *Diagnostic Testing,* she suspected
what she would find when she opened to the places
marked by the yellow slips.

And there they were. Examples of the kinds of tests
administered by Herbert Gray. Inkblots, diagrams of
puzzles—a wooden elephant, fragments of birds to be
reassembled—and a whole chapter on the Thematic
Apperception Test, listing the pictures that would be
shown to the subject for his reactions: woman standing at window, man staring at her; two children playing in yard . . .

Of course, the text also discussed the purpose and
logic of the exercises—with sample responses described, a whole range of responses, from those that
established serious mental disorder to those considered clinically normal, acceptable.

To study these texts, Carol realized, was to know
how to face a battery of psychological tests and create
the picture of a personality, one that fell in a category
you could call normal.

He had prepared.

All at once the book in her hands was too heavy to
hold. It seemed to take inordinate strength to close
it, put it back on the table.

"Tommy . . . ," she whispered to herself, as though
invoking his name could call him out of hiding in the
middle of a childish game, bring him smiling before
her to proclaim that he was nothing more than what
she saw.

Tommy. The name, and the guilt attached to it, the insane atrocities, the hideous images of the victims, the memory of Margot and Anne—a whole universe of horror for which he was both god and devil—all of it crowded inside her brain, pushing out the last chance for hope.

She turned away from the table, preparing to leave. And just then a faint sound came rising up the stairwell from the ground floor. The sound of a door closing.

Someone had entered the house.

More noises from below—a rustling, then footsteps, slow and deliberate, each one clearly audible on the uncarpeted polished parquet of the first floor. From the heaviness of the tread Carol knew it could not belong to a woman.

Tommy was home.

Frozen in place, she weighed her choices. Stay in hiding . . . or greet him, act the part of cheerful unknowing sister. Her car was parked right outside, anyway. He had to know she was in the house.

But at the thought of confronting him she knew that feigning ignorance would be impossible. And how would he react to her horror and fear? Margot was dead . . . dozens of women had been butchered. Killing was more than a habit for him; it was a need, a reflex. Could anything shield her from his impulse once he knew what she'd discovered?

She could not will herself to face him. Not only fear restrained her, but disgust. And she recognized, too, a stronger emotion, one she could never have imagined feeling toward her brother until this moment. Absolute loathing.

For Tommy? No, this wasn't her brother. It was a monster, inhabiting a familiar and friendly form merely as a disguise.

The sound of footsteps had faded, disappeared. He must have walked through to the rear of the house.

Could she move quickly enough to get away unseen? She stepped toward the door.

And another barely perceptible noise halted her. A creak from the stairs. Listening harder, she heard another. He was climbing the first flight, but slowly, stealthily. To catch her unaware.

She took a quick light step in retreat and glanced around wildly, seeking a weapon. The chair? A book? A pencil to stab him?

The metal gooseneck lamp! It could stun him if she swung it hard enough. She went carefully into a crouch and disconnected the plug from the socket, then picked up the lamp by its base, lofting it over her head as she tiptoed around the corner of a cutback beside the door.

Silence now. He'd reached the bottom of the small flight to the attic, Carol guessed, and had paused to choose direction. Or had he walked along the corridor, entered a bedroom? The second floor was carpeted everywhere; she wouldn't have heard his movements.

It came from not far away—a slight padding sound. The sole of a shoe laid on the bottom step leading to the attic.

A creak.

Another footstep.

Very slowly Carol arched the lamp over her head, then stood motionless, every muscle aching with the strain of holding her position.

He was still coming. Four more steps. Now she noticed a change in the light as the frame of the open door was blocked by a figure. And then he came forward, crossing toward the table, hand, arm, shoulder creeping into her sightline. Carol tensed to swing down as his head appeared—

Edged by the brim of a homburg.

The shock alone checked her, and the abrupt shift of balance caused her to rock back with a loud bump against the wall. Miller whirled. Seeing Carol with her arm still raised, he threw his hand up to ward off a blow.

Her arm dropped to her side. "I thought you were him," she murmured.

Miller took a deep breath. "Thank God you're all right. When I saw your car out front, I thought maybe he'd been here—or still was, that maybe . . ." He trailed off.

She eyed him suspiciously. "What brought you?"

His heavy shoulders moved under the overcoat. "Same as you, I'd guess. Looking for Tommy. Wanting to end it. You know now, don't you, Carol?"

Escaping from his demanding gaze, she crossed to the table and put the lamp down. "He memorized the tests," she said, keeping her back to Miller. "He knew exactly what to tell the psychiatrist so he would look—"

"He's smart," Miller cut in, his voice low and flat. "A kind of genius. We always knew he had to be."

The plain acceptance of what she had found so startling roused her again to remember that Miller, too, had lies to explain. She spun to face him.

"And you . . . are you any less mad? Any less evil? How can I believe anything you tell me? All you've done is lie." Her voice rose to an impassioned cry. "Why, Paul? Why did everything have to be a lie? Even about your daughter." She advanced on him. "And those records of Frank's. You said they'd clear Tommy, you told me you were taking them to the police. Nothing, nothing you've told me was true. So how can I believe you about my brother—even what I see with my own eyes?" She glanced at the books on the table, threw out her arm, pointed. "How do I know you didn't set this up?"

Miller took off his hat and walked to the center of the attic. "Do you really think I planted them?" He nodded toward the books. "Or do you know that

Tommy's instinct to save himself is almost as strong as his urge to kill. He was buying time, that's all, try-ing—with that part of himself that still wants to stay free—to fool the experts. Trying every way he could to go on looking innocent, doing it with the same care, the same genius, he applies to murder. He hired Frank knowing a time might come when he'd need to set up a screen. He planned his killings to match the pattern of Frank's trips—easy enough since Frank worked for him, and he either knew the business being transacted, or could send Frank where he wanted him to go. Then, of course, Tommy monkeyed with all the travel logs to make the patterns coincide more. And finally, when Margot Jenner left Frank Matheson's apartment after looking for evidence, Tommy intercepted her and killed her—took her out to the deep woods some-where—a last futile attempt to throw the guilt onto his personally selected scapegoat."

Carol could hear Tommy's voice in her head, the echo of the conversation in which Tommy had pro-tested Margot's plan. "And the blood in Frank's car?" she said softly—not arguing, only needing him to ex-plain.

"Like everything else Frank told the police, it's just what he said it was. Blood tests that spilled. For all we know, Tommy provided him with some faulty sample tubes, intending them to leak, leave one more false clue."

Carol didn't challenge him. She still felt almost too weak to stand, slightly dizzy. She bowed her head over the table, praying that some strength would flow back into her body. "Why?" she asked quietly, one word to ask a thousand questions, eulogize the scores of dead, plead the truth from Miller. Why? she meant to ask once more as she turned to him.

But suddenly even the strength to form the word was too much. She was aware of Miller looking back at her strangely, and then, as if through a mist, she saw him lunge forward with his arms outstretched. In the next second she felt herself sliding away down a long shaft into a cavern of nothingness.

33 RETURNING TO CONSCIOUSNESS, she found herself lying on the beige suede sofa in Tommy's living room. A cool, damp cloth was folded across her forehead, and Miller was sitting erect and watchful in a chair nearby. He had taken off his overcoat to spread over her as a blanket, and she could see that he was dressed in a dark blue pinstripe suit, the trousers sharply creased—as if getting near the end of the case was an occasion to be recognized by some formality. As she stirred, he leaned toward her, and as soon as she started to sit up, he held out his hand.

"Stay there awhile longer," he said, his firm manner enough to make her lie back again. "Sometimes the things you know can bring you down as hard as if you were hit by a tree." She rolled her head away toward the back of the couch, not to look at him. Yes, now she knew. And yet the moment her mind was awake again, all she could think of were the untidy loose ends of logic, all the things that still argued against Tommy's guilt. "My friend Anne," she murmured. "Tommy had no reason to kill her, not the way he would with Margot—to protect himself. And you said, right at the beginning, that knowing Anne was in his favor . . . because the killer always chose his victims at random."

"Coincidences are also part of random events," Miller replied. "One night when Tommy went prowling, he chose the university where Anne worked as his hunting ground. And she happened to be the one who crossed his path. Or maybe she was merely the exception that proves the rule. Maybe he harbored some old hatred, and he couldn't control it anymore. As long as he'd become so good at murder, he decided to settle a score."

No, Anne had never hurt Tommy. It couldn't have been vengeance, Carol decided. Just coincidence.

But how odd, she thought then, that she had begun to accept his guilt. He could be a monster, an insane destroyer of anonymous lives encountered at random. But she refused to believe he would have used murder as a tool of vengeance.

She felt herself going mad with the strain of fitting these facts into a new reality. Did it really matter how or why or when or how many times her brother had committed murder? Tommy was the Deep Woods Killer.

An animal wail rose from Carol's lips, and she turned her mouth into the cushions to stifle it. Then she felt Miller's hand laid comfortingly on her back. She bolted up, as if touched by a red-hot iron.

"No! Don't touch me!" she roared savagely as she swung her legs down to the floor. "You're no better than he is, you wear the same false face!"

"I've had my reasons," he said, shaking his head as though in mild reproof of a child's petulant outburst. "Carol, I need your help. I came here looking for Tommy. I've made a habit lately of passing by his house every few days. Yesterday I saw it was standing empty, so I came in . . . and I found the books, the proof he'd studied for the tests. I came back today hoping to find him home, to bring him in. But he's still not here. So obviously he's been away somewhere. If you know where he is, any place we might catch up with him, please don't hold it back. If he's coming here, if you came here to meet him, then say so."

She glared back. "I won't tell you," she said with icy

finality. "Not until I hear your goddamn confession first."

He eyed her coldly and said nothing.

"I need to know why you never told me the truth," she persisted. "You never had to lie to me, that's why I don't understand. I would have trusted you. I *did* trust you. But you never stopped lying, using me. Why, Paul, if you ever cared at all—don't let me wonder forever."

He hesitated another long moment, then rose from the chair and paced to the center of the room. When he started to speak, his voice was so low she could only just hear him; it was the first time his undertone of firm authority was absent.

"Maybe I would have done it differently if you weren't right—if the evil wasn't in me, too. But I knew it was there long before I started looking for this killer. And I knew something else: how hard it was to believe that someone close to you could do this . . . be this kind of animal." He turned back to her. "I always believed Tom was the one. By the time I came to you, I'd been on this case almost five years—not two or three as I once told you. I started working on it as soon as there were half a dozen victims, enough to know the murderer was a serial killer. I'd done enough footwork and backtracking and surveillance to feel it could only be one of three or four men on the list.

"And I had my gut instinct; more than anything else, that told me it was probably Tommy. But he was always clean as a whistle, so clean that of course I kept thinking I must have it wrong, and I kept following other leads. I was just one man, I couldn't stay on top of him all the time." Miller walked to the rear windows, looked out over the pleasant lawn behind the house. "By the time I came to you, I was ready to try anything to break through. If it was Tommy, I thought, perhaps I'd get to him somehow through you. But I knew it wouldn't work if I walked in right at the beginning and told you my suspicions. Even when I did break them gently—one man on a long list, remember—you couldn't accept it. So I did whatever was necessary to get close, little by little, and to prepare you to accept the unacceptable. I had to work on your perceptions, you see, make you doubt the most solid truth, put your mind in a state where everything was open to question—"

"My drawing!" she blurted suddenly. "You went into my apartment and erased one of my sketches." Only now, only in the context of what Miller was saying, did it begin to make sense.

"Yes," he said, "I wanted you to feel unsafe, that was part of it. And I wanted you to share my fears, and know I shared yours. That's why I told you I had a daughter who was a victim—not just to prey on your sympathy, but so you'd feel I was suffering because of this case, just as you were. And having Suzanne for my own made me likable, didn't it, made me noble for pursuing her killer?"

"It started with the book," Carol intoned, working it out for herself as she spoke. "A child's book, so I'd be more touched by your loss." She felt dazed by the callousness of Miller's strategy.

"Yes—Suzanne's book."

"But Mr. Lumley—"

"An old friend. We used to work together."

"In the security business?" she asked, always testing the bounds of his truth.

"Farther back." Miller turned from the window. "I was a military man once. George and I were both with Army Intelligence." He walked toward her slowly. "I was pretty sure you'd want to go looking for me, pick up on that little tag in the back of the book. It was set up so you'd get steered to George. He was ready to help because he knew how desperately I needed to solve this case."

Carol felt shaken again by the idea that he was an

impostor. Was he going to tell her now there was some matter of military security involved in his investigation?

Ignoring her baldly skeptical glance, Miller went on. "It must sound a little crazy to you—maybe it is. But in the middle of madness, trying to confront it, find the cause, sometimes the only way to keep your bearings is to enter into it yourself. Do you really think, Carol, that you've come to the point of believing your brother is guilty only because you've seen those books upstairs? There's more to the journey than that. You're ready at last to believe that Tom could totally manipulate your perception of the real and right, for so long, for so many years, because you had the first lesson from me: it isn't that hard to fool a good heart. There is no truth, not mine, not Tommy's. I wasn't the man you thought I was . . . and neither is he."

He had walked almost to the sofa, was standing over her. The pose was intimidating, as if he were challenging her to keep pressing for answers. But she would not back down. She stood up and looked directly in his eyes. "He's not a mystery anymore. But you're still trying to keep your secrets."

He turned aside. She moved around to face him again. "What did you mean," she asked, "about your friend from the Army helping because he knew how much you needed to solve this?"

She held his gaze, and after a second his lips parted slightly as though he meant to speak. But then she saw a shadow of pain dim his eyes, and he started to turn away. She clutched his shoulder and pulled him back.

"Tell me, goddamn it!" she pleaded. "I have a right to know."

His head went down in a penitent's pose, and he nodded slowly. Then, clasping her arms in his large hands, he eased her back down onto the sofa. How strange, she thought, that she felt no fear of him.

He walked a few steps away after she was seated, and

before he spoke his hands circled in the air—like the nervous pantomime of an actor in rehearsal, Carol thought, speaking lines first in his head. Yet, perhaps for this very reason, she knew that this time it would not be a performance. Telling lies, Miller's delivery had always been flawless. It was only the truth he had to rehearse.

He rubbed a hand once more over his sandy hair and began, looking off toward a corner of the room, looking at nothing but the past. "For a lot of the time I was in the Army, I was stationed in Germany. That was the early sixties, mostly. The wall in Berlin hadn't been up long, there was plenty of bad blood between the East and West—a lot to keep a career intelligence officer busy. So I made my home there, met a lovely German woman, married her and had a son. We were all there right through '71. Then Hanna—my wife—and I decided it was time to leave Berlin. She'd always wanted to live in America. So we came back. I stayed with the service awhile longer, realized that the life we wanted—Hanna wanted, anyway—wasn't affordable on a major's pay, and I left to start the security business. It went well right from the beginning." He glanced down and shook his head, as though regretting that quick success. "We had everything, the good life. And Gary, my son, he took to it all like a prince of the realm. High school football hero, life of the party, always a pretty girl riding next to him in a Corvette he bought as a wreck and fixed up—wouldn't let me get him a new one. And on top of it all, every year, he'd hit for an A in four out of five subjects. There was nothing that kid couldn't do. Nothing," Miller added, his voice falling momentarily to a near whisper.

He turned toward the window again, and as the light caught him in profile, Carol saw his eyes sparkle with an unusual intensity, like very deep, flat water reflecting a high sun. "But he didn't want to go on to college. Could have gotten in anywhere, but he said he wanted to pick up where I'd left off—make a career of the Army and get into the intelligence end, hopefully in Germany. Wanted the excitement, he said, and he was pretty well equipped for it. He'd been eleven when we moved back from abroad, and he'd kept the language, perfectly bilingual. Of course, intelligence work wasn't what his mother and I preferred, but we didn't stand in the way. He enlisted for four years, went through the first year at grunt level, and then got the posting he wanted. U.S. Forces in Germany. He was there another two years and seemed perfectly happy." Miller turned to Carol again. "And from the first year he was there, until they finally stopped him, Gary, my son, my only child, was committing murder. Women he met and charmed on his weekend leaves and furloughs. Women from towns as far as two hundred miles from his base. Two the first year, six the second, eight the third. . . ."

Those newspapers in his house, Carol thought. The ones from Germany. She stared at him, though with the glare of the sunlit window behind him, he was only a dark shape, his face in shadow. But she could tell from his voice, trembling and hoarse with emotion, that he was struggling to retain his composure.

"Of course, we never knew a thing about it—I mean, not even from the news. It wasn't covered here. Oh, I think we learned later there'd been a piece in *Newsweek* about the Germans trying to deal with this unsolvable case. But at the time . . . nothing. The letters he wrote home were, well, like letters you might get from your brother. News of a promotion, observations about the towns he visited. Later it was possible to match up the towns with victims. But not then. We knew nothing. Although it was getting worse . . . because, as I told you, it always does. In the first ten months of the fourth year alone, he killed twelve times. And then . . ." Miller paused and squared his shoulders, a movement oddly like bringing himself to attention, as a military man might to receive either an honor or a reprimand. Then he continued, pushing the words out faster. "For a couple years he'd been able to get back to the States for the holidays. But this time his mother went over. Hanna still had family there, her mother and a married sister. She stayed with them in Stuttgart a few days, then went up to visit with Gary at his base in Mainz. Four days before Christmas, they found Hanna with her throat cut in the hotel where she was staying. In another room down the hall was another victim, bludgeoned to death. He went absent without leave after that, which broke the case open. I don't think there's been a bigger manhunt in Germany, but he managed to stay on the loose for another day and a night, killed two more times, one of them a girl of fourteen. Then they got him, tried him, put him in a prison for the criminally insane. He's still there."

He came back to the chair next to her and slumped down, chin on his chest, eyes down. During the brief time his face had been in shadow, it seemed to Carol to have aged years.

"But it didn't end there," he said wearily. "Not for me. I couldn't work—wasn't good for a thing, in fact. I'd sit all day and think about it, lie awake all night. How could this child of mine do such things? What was there in me to produce such evil? What . . . ?" He paused, silently asking the questions yet again.

"But there weren't any answers, not in my mind, not in the safe little hiding place I'd made for myself. So I decided to go into his world, his mind—by trying to understand another serial murderer. That's when I set out to find the Deep Woods Killer." He brought his eyes up to meet Carol's. "I know I'm obsessed by the need to understand. I know I've gone about it in a bad way at times. But nothing else matters, nothing but trying to scrape one more handful of human comprehension out of all the blood and misery."

He fell silent. For a long time, perhaps a couple of minutes, Carol watched him sitting with his head down, gazing at the floor. She kept waiting for him to continue, feeling there was one thing more she had to know, and that he would surely raise it without being asked. But he didn't. And though she was moved by his tragedy, she felt anger building at the way it had led him to brutalize her own life, deal with her in a way that left a wound no less deep if less bloody than the slash of a killer's blade.

Finally, fighting to keep the emotion out of her voice, she had to ask. "And when you made love to me, was that also part of the strategy?"

His head came up sharply, though the reply was another long moment in coming. "It was wrong of me." Then he stood up. "Now you've had my confession. So let's find Tommy. Tell me where you think he might be."

His cool words only gouged the wound deeper. As she looked at him now, hatred flared in her. She rose to her feet slowly, while the burning of an inner fire of rage rose up through her belly into her brain.

"So that's all," she said, holding her voice low only with the most ferocious determination. "Let's go and find him. Nothing more to say. It was wrong of you and that's it. You did whatever you had to do to *me*— used *me*, even made love to me—on the chance I might give you one clue, one insight, to hunt down a killer . . . and that's all you can say?"

"Whatever it took to find him, I had to do. And I still need you, Carol. Because the evidence we have on Tommy now—the indications that the psych tests were a fraud—that isn't enough to convict him. We may know what it means, but it won't stand in a court of law, not if he doesn't confess. So if there's anything else you can think of—"

She couldn't let him finish before the fury finally

spewed out. She rushed at him, shouting, "You bastard, you unholy bastard, I could kill you."

She raised her fists to pummel at his face, but he caught her by the wrists and held on until the strength in her arms ebbed, and the will to hurt him died.

"I'm sorry, Carol," he said as he let go, "believe me I'm sorry. But this killer had to be stopped."

"Which killer?" she snarled. "The one you've been looking for was never my brother. You were looking for the killer in yourself, Paul. And where he lives in you is in caring so precious little about what you do to people—did to me—to get what you want."

He regarded her thoughtfully a moment, then he went to the sofa, picked up his overcoat, and slipped it on.

"Are you going to tell me where he is, Carol? Tommy's on the run now, the frenzy could explode anytime. Several lives could be riding on what you do."

The last of the anger went out of her. Only sadness was left. Whatever he'd been wrong about, Carol knew, he was right that she could no longer protect Tommy without making innocent people pay the price.

"He went to Vermont," she said quietly. "His wife's there with her parents in Rutland, and he wanted to see her one more time."

"One more," Miller repeated. "He said that?"

Carol shrugged. "I don't know, I don't remember. None of what he said seems to matter anymore. But he was driving back today. I thought he'd be coming here first."

Miller nodded, then swept a glance around and moved to the phone, visible through the opening to the living room, on a table in the library.

Carol stood by as he made a call—to the task force, she realized, when she heard him ask for Elward Daley.

"Daley," he said in a moment, talking very fast.

"This is Paul Miller. I'm certain that Warren's the one. From the look of things, he's on the edge, moving around a lot. Went up to Vermont, and now he's on the way back. I thought it might be worth covering the roads from Rutland to—"

Miller stopped suddenly, evidently cut off by Daley. Carol saw his expression tighten and the blood drain from his face. "When was that?" he asked.

He got his answer, said a quick good-bye, and cradled the phone. Before Carol could ask what had happened, he said, "Where else might he go, Carol? If he didn't come here . . . where else?"

She didn't have to ask him why, after all. The straining urgency in his voice told her all she needed—wanted—to know.

Even as she answered his question without hesitation, she was wondering if anything might have been different if she hadn't insisted on extracting a confession of her own.

34 AT THE HOUSE ON LLOYD'S NECK ROAD, only a black Chevy hatchback and an old Jeep were parked in the driveway. No sign of Tommy's silver Nissan.

"He's not here," Carol said.

"Whose cars are those?" Paul asked.

"It must be the people from the auctioneer—the appraisers. They had a key."

In a reckless two-hour journey, speeding the entire way, Paul had driven to Pete Warren's house. Carol's fractured mind had dwelled on the surface—on the miracle of not being stopped and given a ticket, on the sheer blue plate of sky broken only by two twisting strands of cloud. Even when Paul related his conversation with the police, his voice came to her as though he were calling out from the depths of a canyon. Just past six o'clock this morning, the police had told him, a nurse had arrived home at her apartment in Huntington. She had been the lucky one, had spent the night with her boyfriend only a few blocks away. While she slept, an intruder had entered the apartment where she lived and brutally attacked her four roommates, all nurses, asleep in their beds. Three were dead. Whether the fourth would live was still in doubt.

At the front stoop of her father's house Carol glanced over her shoulder, hoping against hope that Tommy would show up, and then at the same instant praying he wouldn't. It chilled her to think he would yet round the bend at the bottom of the hill, park in the driveway, step out smiling—a picture of innocence.

The front door was unlocked. In the entrance hall to the living room Carol saw two men sitting on the roll-arm couch, clipboards in their hands, and stacks of oaktag tickets with strings scattered on the floor.

"You must be Miss Warren," one of them said, standing. He introduced himself, but Carol didn't quite get the name—Norton or Norman or something like that. He said they had been labeling the furniture for an hour. "We're just about done, ma'am."

"Take your time," Carol said blankly.

Paul settled himself by the bay window. "I'll wait here," he said.

Watching for Tommy, Carol thought. What would he do if Tommy did arrive?

By now every object in the house had been tagged with a price. Recalling Tommy's request to keep his mementos, Carol climbed the stairs to his room. Methodically she untacked high school baseball pennants from the sloping dormered wall and piled them on the bed. Every time she heard a car motor she darted to the window and peered out.

Finally the appraisers departed, and she was left facing Paul, alone, in the living room.

"He's not coming, Carol. He's on the run."

"So what will you do?"

"Keep hunting, try to get to him before he does it again. I'm going to Huntington now, I want to see the place where those nurses were killed."

For a second she felt it was careless of Paul to remind her of the bloody crime. Then she realized he had chosen his words deliberately, underscoring the evil of complicity if she were to keep any secrets that might help apprehend Tommy sooner.

"I'll stay here," she said. "He still might come."

"You can't stay alone. It isn't safe. I want you with me."

To see an apartment where several women had been slaughtered? Carol recalled the day she had forced Eric to take her downtown, allowed herself to view the photographs of dead women, as if they might relinquish a secret, prove Tommy's innocence, offer her an escape from the nightmare.

Could she still hope to uncover such a secret?

Or did she need a different kind of discovery? Could she escape from this nightmare only by walking through its dark, bloody center? Could she ever know the truth of what Tommy was—the truth of her own flesh—if she did not see the absolute reality of his crime?

"I'll get my coat," she said.

It was an afternoon at the circus.

All around them were red lights flashing, blue barricades, television crews doing balancing acts with cameras on their shoulders. But the ringmasters wore no bright red uniforms here. They wore drab gray overcoats with badges flapping from their breast pockets.

Carol trailed behind Paul through a crowd of onlookers up to the sidewalk, where a cordon blocked the way. At the top of a small rising lawn was a three-story house of fake rusticated stucco. Low evergreen bushes lined the path to the porch. As Paul reached the sawhorse barricade, a tall woman in an orange parka and black slacks started down the steps. She squeezed between the sawhorses and headed for Paul as if she knew him. With her long dark hair and the wire-rim glasses on her young, sweet face, she seemed incongruous to Carol, and when she lifted her arm to wave away two men running toward her, she looked like a school crossing guard who had roamed here by mistake.

"Hi, Miller."

"Hello, Diane." Paul made introductions. "Carol,

this is Diane Monroe, she's a Suffolk County police detective, a friend of mine. Diane, this is Carol Warren."

"Warren?" the policewoman said.

Carol caught the shocked, harsh glare that came with the recognition of her name. But she didn't flinch. She had already prepared herself, anticipated that for the rest of her life people might recognize her name.

"It's okay, Diane," Paul said. "Trust me. What do you have?"

The woman returned her attention to Paul. "It's spotless. We've been over every inch. So far not a clue. Nothing. Woodsie is freaking, but he still doesn't miss a trick."

"The bodies?" Paul asked.

"Still inside. The M.E. doesn't want us to move them yet."

Their language had the feeling of a private code, Carol thought. Cold and precise, with a peculiar detachment.

"The fourth girl," Paul went on.

"Coma," the woman said.

"Any chance . . . ?"

"Less than even," Diane Monroe replied in a dispirited tone. "We've got two guys waiting by her bed just in case, but I wouldn't count on getting anything from her."

"Okay," Paul said, "give me a pass."

The woman reached into her pocket and pulled out a pink card, scribbled Paul's name on it.

"Carol, wait here for me."

"No," Carol said.

Paul laid a gloved hand on her shoulder. "Carol, you don't want to see—"

"No," she repeated, her voice hard. She had not come with Paul to stand aside, guarded by a wilderness of lights and cars and blue-suited policemen. She looked directly at the detective. "Give me a pass, please."

The woman glanced toward Paul. He nodded, and she slowly retrieved another pink card from her pocket. For a moment she held her pen, peering over the top of her glasses. "Want me to put 'Warren' on this?" she asked.

"That's my name," Carol said.

Diane Monroe filled out the pink card and slid the barricade back to let them pass.

Inside the house, in the cramped first-floor hallway, dozens of uniformed policemen jostled against photographers. At first it seemed to be a mad rush of people battling for ground, and then Carol realized it was only in her mind. Despite the closeness, and the narrow space packed tight as a subway car, the teams of police technicians went about their business. Three white-coated men knelt on the floor, scraping a dingy blue carpet with tweezers and brushes. By the stairs, a slender bald man in a tan leisure suit held a small aerosol can, shooting sprays of fine powder onto the banister.

Carol had started for the stairs when she saw Eric Gaines coming toward her.

"Oh, Carol . . . ," he said sympathetically, and put his arms around her. She stood motionless for a second, unable to return his embrace, then rested her head against his chest.

"How did you get here?" he asked.

She pulled away and gestured toward Paul. "Eric, you know Paul Miller, don't you?"

"We talked once," he said with a narrow smile.

Carol remembered then that Eric had questioned Paul after arresting him.

Eric went on: "You could've saved everybody a lot of trouble, Mr. Miller, if you'd worked with us in the first place."

"Of course, Lieutenant," Paul said with caustic irritation. "Though perhaps you're not aware of my efforts to provide you jokers with a lead two years ago to . . . to the right man. As I remember the situation now, the task force relegated it to the garbage."

"Ease up," Eric said sharply. "That was before I worked there, they hadn't even geared up yet, and you could've come back. How the hell were we supposed to know you were on the level? If you'd cooperated a little—"

"Never mind now," Paul said. "We all could have handled ourselves better."

He started toward the second floor, and Carol moved to follow. But before she reached the first step, Eric blocked her path.

"Carol, you can't," he said in a low voice. "It's rough up there."

"I'll be all right," Carol said evenly.

"You're not hearing me, Carol, it's . . . a slaughterhouse, worse than you can imagine."

. . . just how bad . . .

Ed Donaldson's words floated into her mind. How long ago had Anne's father admitted his anguish at allowing his wife to identify their daughter's body? That had happened in another life, Carol thought. Whoever she had been then would not have climbed these stairs.

"I'm going up, Eric."

The very determination in her words seemed to push him out of her path.

"I wish I could stop you," he said.

"Me, too," she said. "But no one can."

Carol climbed the steps behind Eric, who talked over his shoulder to Paul. The killer, he explained, had entered through a second-floor bedroom window. "He gagged the girl in the first room, then he raped her. Or maybe he killed her first, we don't know yet. He did the second one the same way. Then he tied up the third and fourth victims . . . dragged them across the hall and then did them in the same room. So one of them was watching. No witnesses yet unless the girl in the hospital . . ."

They had reached the top of the stairway. Eric pushed the door open, and Carol saw a streak of red along the yellow wall to her right. Ahead of her a floodlamp was shining into a room. More men were crawling on the carpeting, holding small brushes; a score of others milled around looking oddly like shoppers browsing in a store.

She edged past them. Busy with their own tasks, none noticed her. She felt a hand brush her arm and turned to see Eric shaking his head, again trying to persuade her not to look. But she moved straight past him, too, and stopped behind the tripod holding the lamp. And as she peered over the metal bowl of its shade, her eyes registered a single bloodied arm. Now the rest came—at first dimly and in flashes, and then it spread out onto a flat canvas, a painting: the pool of blood like the symbol on a flag, white sheets gathered on the bed, a woman's thighs, her arched back and arms roped to the posts of a chair, her breasts falling over the top, a brown plastic object inserted between her legs, the head slumped forward, white cloth tied through her mouth, her feet twisted and splayed in blood.

For a single second Carol stood motionless, heard a voice—"It's a miracle nobody saw him, he must've been covered from head to foot, every inch of him"—and then she knew she had seen too much. She ran down the hall but got only as far as the top of the stairs before she began to retch. And when her stomach was done churning she let them carry her down, Paul on one side with his arm around her waist, Eric on the other with her arm slung over his shoulder.

Outside, they sat her on a porch step. She wiped her face and on Paul's instructions took deep breaths to the count of ten.

The woman detective who had provided the passes was hurrying up the steps. She took one look at Carol, another at Eric and Paul. "Assholes," she snapped. "What the hell did you let her up there for?" She thrust a long strip of paper at Paul. "New York Telephone finally came through."

Paul studied the sheet. "I thought so," he muttered.

Carol lifted her head. "What is it?"

"A list of phone calls made from Margot Jenner's apartment the afternoon she disappeared."

Carol stood up expectantly.

"She called your brother," Paul went on. "She was on the line with him for seven minutes. She must have told him what she was going to do."

"Or asked him for help," Carol said, instantly realizing that although she had meant to exonerate Tommy by casting Margot's call in an innocent light, she had done exactly the opposite. She remembered Tommy's adamant demand that Margot not get involved, and Margot must have called to convince him, or to ask his permission.

Whatever the interpretation, Tommy had known where Margot would be. And he could have followed her, could have been there even before Frank. . . .

Carol walked away as the conversation between Paul and the detectives continued. She turned at the bottom of the steps, out onto the hill above the street. The television cameramen still swarmed, the dome lights on the police cars were still flashing. Moving as if under water, she drifted around to the side of the house, away from the chaos. It was quieter here. She found a metal guard railing above the cement stairs leading to the basement and balanced herself on it. The touch of the cool metal on her legs felt soothing.

Raised voices stole her moment of tranquillity: "And that's how he got in. Why the hell didn't anybody see him?"

" 'Cause nobody's awake at four fucking o'clock in the morning, that's why."

Carol turned toward the voices, coming from farther back on the lawn. Several men were gathered under an old maple tree with an elaborate structure of branches. She could see the condensation of their breath faintly visible in the chilly air.

"Gettin' in that window is a lotta fuckin' work," one of the men said. "Why not a ladder?"

"What would you carry?" another voice asked. "A ladder, or rope? I mean, what fits in a car?"

So Tommy . . . no, the killer . . . the killer had climbed a tree to reach the second-floor window. Propelled by curiosity—or was it intuition?—Carol walked closer. A last dim shaft of fading sunlight illuminated a strand of heavy white cord hanging almost to the ground. And then, as Carol's eyes traveled up the rope, she saw how it was secured to the branch. One knot over another, a clump of knots tied within each other, around each other.

As if done by a child, Carol thought, who wasn't sure it would hold.

In the car Paul reached over and gently touched her cheek.

"You're tired," he said.

She removed his hand with hers, said nothing, and just stared through the windshield. Am I like him? she wondered. How much of the killer is in me, in my blood?

"We have to stop him," she said at last.

"What is it?" Paul asked. "What made the penny drop? The books in his house?"

"The rope," she said quietly. And then she explained. It was done exactly like the one Tommy had tied to the tree in their backyard fairy-tale kingdom. Knotted over and over and over. "Did he think I'd see it?" Carol asked. "Maybe he left it as a clue for me."

"Carol, his mind wouldn't work that way, there isn't a chance he'd think—"

"But why not?" she asked, desperate to believe that there was one atom of decency in Tommy, that he was begging to be stopped, crying out for *her* help. "It's the only reason. The only reason to tie the rope that way is to let me know. He might guess you'd bring me here." She grabbed Paul's hand. "I'd testify to what it means. I really would."

"If only that were enough," Paul said. With all they had learned about Tommy, he pointed out, and even with Carol's willingness to add her own belief to the record, the real evidence constituted nothing more than wisps of smoke.

"Those knots may clinch it for you," he said, "but it's not proof. Not for a jury. If we find him now, if he's not halfway across the country getting ready to kill again, and if he offers us one minuscule shred of evidence, a good lawyer could still raise reasonable doubt. If Tommy keeps up his unshakable facade, who knows what a jury would do?" Paul rested his palms against the steering wheel and continued in a dry, pitiless tone. "They had circumstantial evidence on my son from the German police, but all the Army thought about was the political damage, the guilt of an American soldier, and when they said he was insane, the Army demanded that he be put in a military prison. I don't know what he's capable of. Maybe someday he'll convince them he's sane, maybe he'll get out . . . and kill again."

"And Tommy?" Carol said. "You think a jury will acquit him?"

Paul shrugged. "You can never be sure. Though maybe something from the past will come out, evidence nobody's found yet."

He started the car, backed out past the police cordon.

"Are you taking me home?" Carol asked.

"To your father's house," Paul said.

"You don't think Tommy would still—"

"He came this way, and it's nearby. Maybe you're right—maybe he wanted to leave a clue. Maybe there's a part of him that wants it to end."

IN THE
DEEP
WOODS

He pushed the door open very slowly and stood for a long moment at the threshold, listening.

Hi, anybody home?

In the silence, he could hear the echo of his younger voice from hundreds of past homecomings. But today's was like no other, of course. It would be his last. No point in coming home anymore.

He waited another second, decided the house was empty, and then stepped in and closed the door behind him. With a wrapped bouquet of flowers tucked under his arm while he held on to a small satchel, and his shoes—removed before he had climbed the porch steps—dangling from his other hand, he was aware of looking like some cartoon of an errant, apologetic husband sneaking in after hours.

But he'd never been a sneak, never meant to be. Keeping secrets was different from being sneaky. Hadn't she once assured him of that herself? So much of what he remembered about her was hazy—but there did seem to be a time long ago when he hadn't been able to sleep, and he'd tiptoed around and come upon her sitting naked in front of a mirror, moaning, her head thrown back. She had scolded him, said it was bad to go sneaking around, but then she had lifted him onto her lap and hugged him and cooed in his ear, "It's all right for us to have our little secrets, my darling. . . ."

Now, in the gloom of late afternoon, he could almost see her, floating toward him, ready to love him no-matter-what. Look at you. Where on earth did you get so filthy? Well, let's get you cleaned up. *As if he had simply come in from playing in a muddy yard.*

Of course, she was right, he had to get cleaned up.

Moving to the kitchen, he took from under his shirt the tightly folded plastic drop cloth that had been spread over the car seat, and set it down with his shoes on the stovetop. Then he pulled several handfuls of paper towels from the roll over the sink and walked over to the laundry alcove. By the washer-dryer he spread the towels in flat strips to form a small protective carpet over the tile floor, and standing in the middle of it, he stripped off all his clothes.

Naked, he headed for the cupboard where the bleach and soaps had always been kept. Suddenly the thought struck that maybe the cupboard was empty. Had any laundry been done here lately? He lunged anxiously for the door of the cupboard, then smiled with relief at the sight of all the boxes and bottles.

Soon he had the washer going, half a bottle of bleach in the water. Then he rolled up the blotchy red paper towels, lit a corner with the flame from the stove, and let them burn in the sink, running water from the tap to wash the charred remnants down the drain. He bunched the plastic drop cloth into the old dish basin and swilled it around in warm, soapy water. He turned on one of the stove burners and held the shoes above it, carefully singeing away anything that was stuck to the soles.

He went upstairs, took a shower, then came back down to the kitchen. Waiting for the wash cycle to finish, he sat naked at the table, half dozing. After pouring in more bleach and starting the washer through a second cycle, he dealt with the flowers. They had wilted from lying in the car, so after standing them in a vase of water, he put the whole arrangement into the refrigerator. He wrote a note to go with the flowers, then dozed while he waited for the second cycle to finish. He couldn't remember ever feeling so tired, but before he could go to bed the clothes had to be dried and folded. Everything neat and in its place.

At last it was all done, and he was able to go up to his room. In one of the drawers of the old dresser, he found a pair of pajamas, and he put them on, then smiled at the view of himself in the mirror on the closet door, arms and legs protruding from shrunken shirt and trousers.

In bed, for a minute before turning out the light, he lay looking up at the ceiling, thinking back over the day. He had been out of control, he realized, stepping much too far over the line. Too much risk. It mustn't ever happen again— though it had ended all right, thank God. He'd done a perfect job of cleaning up, he had a handle on things again. Once he'd had a full night's sleep, he'd be good as new, ready for business-as-usual.

He reached over to the bedside lamp and switched it off. Just before drifting out of consciousness, he saw for a second a girl's face, smiling back at him. But he couldn't remember which one it was.

35

THE STREET RUNNING IN FRONT of the house was eerily quiet and deserted. In two or three of the homes lamplight could be seen shining in the windows, pale pastel squares of yellow against the first hint of evening purple. But at an hour when children were usually still in the yards or taking a last turn on their bikes, when commuters should have been ambling home from the station and older people out walking their dogs, there was no life at all. It was like a news photo of a town left abandoned because of a nuclear meltdown.

As they drove toward her father's house at the middle of the long block, Carol turned to Miller. "Something's happened, Paul," she said. "Where is everybody?"

"They've been told to stay inside or stay away."

"Told . . . ?"

"By the police. I'm sure they went house to house and warned people there might be trouble." He glanced over to her as he began to slow the car. "I steered them here, Carol, in case Tommy turned up. He must have, because the surveillance is in place." As they drove past a dark sedan parked on the street, Miller nodded toward it. Carol noticed the man sitting behind the wheel, saw the tip of his cigarette wink through the gloom.

Carol shook her head. "Why not just . . . arrest Tommy?" It felt strange to be saying a word that ratified her brother's status as a criminal.

"I suggested that they wait," Miller said. He braked the station wagon to a halt. They had arrived at the turn into the driveway where Tommy's silver Nissan stood, blatantly parked at the head.

Miller shut off the ignition, and both he and Carol gazed silently at the car in the drive. The meaning of its presence was clear. Tommy still felt he had nothing to hide.

"It comes back to having so little real evidence," Miller said at last. "We can pull him in, question him forever, but he'll stonewall us. In the end it'll always be a matter of needing proof. Without it, he'll stay free." Miller turned to Carol. "That's why I told the police to hold off until we could get here. Until you could talk to Tommy first."

"And say what, Paul?"

"Whatever it takes to get a confession. You're the only one who has a chance, Carol. This kind of killer may never admit what he's done."

Carol glanced from the car to the house. There were no lights on inside, and as she stared at the blank glass of the bay window, her mind started rapidly replaying scenes that had unfolded behind them long ago, moments of life in that house. Birthday parties, family arguments, holiday gatherings, first dates, ruined dinners, idle memories of times of laughter and sadness. How had they combined to breed a man devoid of any pity or compassion, any comprehension of pain, anything but a hunger to kill?

Or was there just enough of a thread to tie him to humanity—a willingness to acknowledge the monstrous wrong?

"I'll try," she said quietly.

As they got out of the car, Carol saw through the gathering twilight a pair of headlights turn a far corner at one end of Lloyd's Neck Road, and then stop abruptly. It was still light enough to see that the vehicle was a large police van and it was positioned to block the street. Turning in the other direction, Carol saw that a couple of police cars had performed the same maneuver at the other intersection.

"You go in first, quietly," Paul murmured to her as they approached the steps. "I'll follow and cover you . . . but, if possible, talk to him without his knowing I'm around."

They walked softly up to the door. As Carol took the key out of her bag, Miller stepped to one side and drew a revolver from a shoulder holster. Carol stared at it resentfully.

"You won't need that, Paul."

"Probably not. But we don't know yet why he's inside with all the lights out, and I'd rather be ready than dead. Now," he ordered flatly, "open the door."

Carol slipped the key in the lock and pushed the door back noiselessly. "Should I turn on a light?" she asked.

"Go in the way you would normally."

Carol reached around the frame, felt for the switch, and flipped it on. Light from an old brass ceiling fixture shone down the empty front hall. In the bright blaze Carol's eyes were drawn at once to the vase of fresh yellow tulips that stood on a table at the side. Propped up against the vase was a piece of notepaper. At a gesture from Miller, Carol walked across the threshold into the house and went to pick up the note. She read the words, handwritten in steady, even lines:

> Hi, Carrie! Sorry I couldn't make it back earlier. It didn't work out with Jill, but I gave it the old college try. Had a little car trouble on the drive down from Vt. and arrived here bushed, so I hit the hay and I'll see you in the A.M. We'll go visit Dad together, okay? Love you,
>
>   T

Against the background of all she knew now, the
cheerful note and the bright gift of flowers were bizarre. Carol felt her equilibrium so thrown off-center
that a wave of nausea passed through her.

She swallowed hard and passed the note to Paul,
who had closed the door softly behind him.

As he was reading, Carol became aware of the odor
suffusing the air around her, a pungent, somewhat me-
tallic odor that seemed to emanate from the rear of
the house. She looked toward the darkened doorway
of the kitchen, then took a step.

Instantly Paul reached out and clutched her shoulder, holding her back. From the way he had his head
lifted, his nostrils flared, Carol could see he was also
disturbed by the smell. He moved around to precede
her, his gun still drawn as they edged into the kitchen,
and Carol pulled the string of an overhead fluorescent
fixture.

Bathed in harsh light, the kitchen stood clean and
empty, a housekeeper's dream. The odor was stronger
here; even before Carol saw the accordion door folded
open, revealing the alcove where a washing machine
and dryer were installed, she had identified the odor
as strong laundry bleach. Paul dropped the gun into
his pocket as he moved to the alcove, Carol behind
him. Atop the dryer sat a low pile of folded clothes,
only a few items. Paul shuffled through them, unfold-
ing each, and holding them up for examination: a
plain white shirt, white underwear and socks, and a
pair of jeans that had only the palest hint of blue left
in the denim. As Carol moved beside him and took the
shirt to study for herself, she felt a residue of warmth
still radiating from the dryer.

In a low voice Paul said, "They might've been
soaked in blood. We'll never know."

After a second Carol remarked, "The note said he's
gone to sleep."

"Maybe he did. He'd be capable of it."

"His bedroom's upstairs." Carol led Paul out of the kitchen and up to the second-floor landing. She pointed across to Tommy's room, at the end of a short corridor. The door was ajar, showing a thin seam of the darkness within. But the corridor was only dimly visible in the glow rising up the stairwell, and Carol reached to turn on another light.

Miller stayed her hand. "No, it's better like this. I'll wait here. Go in and wake him, leave the door open so I can hear what he says."

Carol squared her shoulders as though it were she who was being called to face a tribunal, and then she walked to the door of Tommy's room. With the flat of her hand she shoved it back, then waited a second as her eyes adjusted. Night had fallen, but a streetlamp outside threw enough ambient light through the window so that she could see Tommy on his bed, lying on his side with his face toward the door. She couldn't be sure, but it seemed that his eyes were closed.

She approached the bed slowly, then switched on the lamp on the low night table. A shaft of harsh illumination fell across his face. For a second the features remained in total repose. So handsome, Carol thought, his future had never been anything but bright. Then his eyes flickered open. He focused on her and smiled.

"Carrie . . . ," he mumbled sleepily.

"Hello, Tommy." She was quaking, unable to keep the tremor from her voice.

He pulled himself up on his elbows and peered at her, trying to see past the lamp's glare. "You okay?"

"No," she whispered, her voice failing, "no, I'm not too well at all."

He sat up, swiped the hair out of his eyes. "Hey, what is it? You sound awful."

"Oh, God, Tommy," she broke into a soft cry, "don't pretend anymore. Please. Make this a little easier, I'm begging you. . . ." She went to her knees right beside him, like a little girl saying her prayers at bed-time.

He looked at her with what appeared to be the most genuine astonishment. "Make what easier?"

"I know. I saw what . . . what you did last night. I know it's you. I know, I know, I know, I know." Repeating it, she felt she was taking some kind of vow, an oath not to be deceived no matter how brilliantly he played his part. "Can't you let it end easily? You're sick, Tommy, so terribly sick."

He threw back the blankets now so that he could sit up fully and grasp her. "Jesus, Sis. What the hell's happened? You're telling me I'm sick, and you're the one talking gibberish."

As he leaned over with concern, Carol met his eyes with hers. "Tell me again, Tommy, keep looking at me and tell me again: you didn't kill Anne . . . or Margot . . . or dozens of other young women you picked up. Tell me again that you aren't the Deep Woods Killer. Just keep looking at me and tell me once more."

She held his gaze rigidly in hers. For a very long time their eyes remained locked, but Tommy said nothing. No shocked denial, no angry denunciation of betrayal. Then his lips twitched slightly, and at last the smile came, his perfectly charming smile.

"Sure, I'll tell you," he said mildly, "if that's what you need to hear. I never killed anyone. Never. Why would I?"

There had to be some way to shake his pose. If she meant anything at all to him. "Tommy. I loved Margot, you know that, loved her very much." She stopped, choked up for a moment as she remembered the pictures she had seen of victims who had lain undiscovered for months, in the wilderness among scavenging animals. "Oh, God, I'm begging you, Tommy, tell me where Margot—where the body is—"

"Hey, Sis," he shrugged ingenuously, "you're way out of line. I didn't do anything."

"Please, Tommy," she went on steadily. "Let my friend . . . let her have a decent burial."

"I can't help you, Carrie," he said in a tone of genuine heartfelt regret. "But why are you even asking? You know where she is—"

"I—?"

"Somewhere in the woods. Isn't that where this guy leaves all his victims? Somewhere deep in the woods . . ."

She might have stopped now. Yet she could not believe the facade would never crack. There must be some test that would defeat him, one fact over which he would stumble.

Then something came to mind. "Tommy, you did a laundry downstairs. Used a lot of bleach, the whole house reeks of it. Why, Tommy? Why would you do that?"

He responded as if there were nothing strange in her shifting so suddenly from accusations of murder to a question about laundry. With a passive shrug he supplied an answer. "Didn't my note say I had car trouble on the drive from Vermont? Got some grease and mud on my clothes. Hard stuff to get out."

"Hard stuff," she echoed in a near whisper.

There was a silence.

"Listen, Carrie," Tommy said blithely after another second. "I don't know what's gone wrong, but I really am totally wiped out. So I'd like to go back to sleep. Could we talk more about this in the morning? I sure would like to straighten it out."

Carol had nothing left. Whatever she could say, she knew beyond doubt, would make no difference. "Sure," she replied.

As Tommy started to recline again, he gave Carol another smile. Then, reaching for the lamp, he paused and tilted his head up in a way obviously mean to invite a sisterly kiss good-night.

Carol's eyes welled with tears as she shook her head slowly from side to side several times, stopping only when the drops began raining down her cheeks. Then she turned and left the room.

Behind her the light clicked off.

Miller was right outside. His nod told Carol that he'd heard and accepted that nothing could be done. Pulling her back along the corridor to the landing, he whispered as softly as possible, barely more than mouthing the words.

"Go down and get the police—just go outside and signal. I'll take care of things up here." Carol looked at him questioningly. "He's got to get up, and dressed, so the police can try for a confession, too."

As she started to descend the stairs, Carol took a last look back and saw Miller hesitate at the door of Tommy's room, then put a hand into his pocket before moving ahead.

She hurried out, and had her foot on the porch step when she heard the sharp report. For a second her mind couldn't grasp what it was. Just the door slamming shut behind her? But the hinges were well-worn, the door always closed softly on its latch.

Then the realization came: his final lie.

"Paul!" she shrieked. "No! NO!"

But as she plunged back toward the closed front door, the second shot came.

Her hands were shaking so badly that she had trouble pulling the key from her purse, and then she couldn't fit it into the lock.

But it didn't matter. Before she could open the door, there were people swarming up the steps and crowding the porch around her, and one of them rammed into the door with his shoulders, busting it open, and then the stream of policemen was flowing past her, jostling her as they proceeded straight up the stairs.

She drifted after them in a daze, until she felt a firm grip on one of her arms. She let herself be pulled around—and saw Eric.

"Not this time, Carol. Save yourself."

She stared back at him. "Tell me what's happened."

Eric nodded and started to dash up the stairs. But he had taken only two steps when a uniformed policeman came from the room to the top of the landing.

"Both of 'em, Lieutenant," the cop called down. "Homicide, suicide."

Eric spun back to Carol. Shattered, she turned from him and stumbled out of the house again.

She stood and looked at the whirl of activity in the street. The circus had become a magic show, cars and trucks and crowds materializing from nowhere, while simultaneously her whole idea of what was real and solid disappeared.

Then Eric was there again, in front of her. He put his arms around her and pulled her into the kind of plain, encompassing embrace that a mountaineer might use to protect a frostbitten companion from a blizzard.

She nestled into it.

A minute or two passed before she found the words. "Will it ever be better again?"

"Maybe not everything," he said. "But some things will." He eased her back slightly and waited until she lifted her face. "That's a promise I could make if you'd let me—some things will."

Carol gave him no answer, merely put her face to his shoulder again, closed her eyes, and kept clinging tightly.

But in the darkness of her mind, the little girl she had guided through every perilous adventure was feeling her way out of the pitch-black cave where the monsters lived, groping along walls so rough they made her hands bleed, while she headed for one infinitely distant pinprick of light.

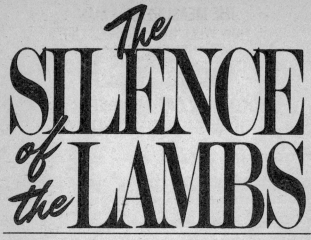

THE SILENCE OF THE LAMBS

THE ELECTRIFYING BESTSELLER BY
THOMAS HARRIS

" THRILLERS DON'T COME ANY BETTER THAN THIS."
— *CLIVE BARKER*

"HARRIS IS QUITE SIMPLY THE BEST SUSPENSE NOVELIST
WORKING TODAY."
— *The Washington Post*

THE MEASURE OF A MAN
IS HOW WELL HE SURVIVES LIFE'S

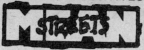

BOLD NEW CRIME NOVELS BY TODAY'S HOTTEST TALENTS

BAD GUYS (July 1989)
Eugene Izzi
———— 91493-8 $3.95 U.S.   ———— 91494-6 $4.95 Can.

CAJUN NIGHTS (August 1989)
D.J. Donaldson
———— 91610-8 $3.95 U.S.   ———— 91611-6 $4.95 Can.

MICHIGAN ROLL (September 1989)
Tom Kakonis
———— 91684-1 $3.95 U.S.   ———— 91686-8 $4.95 Can.

SUDDEN ICE (October 1989)
Jim Leeke
———— 91620-5 $3.95 U.S.   ———— 91621-3 $4.95 Can.

DROP-OFF (November 1989)
Ken Grissom
———— 91616-7 $3.95 U.S.   ———— 91617-5 $4.95 Can.

A CALL FROM L.A. (December 1989)
Arthur Hansl
———— 91618-3 $3.95 U.S.   ———— 91619-1 $4.95 Can.

Publishers Book and Audio Mailing Service
P.O. Box 120159, Staten Island, NY 10312-0004

Please send me the book(s) I have checked above. I am enclosing
$———— (please add $1.25 for the first book, and $.25 for each
additional book to cover postage and handling. Send check or
money order only—no CODs.)

Name _____

Address _____

City _____ State/Zip _____

Please allow six weeks for delivery. Prices subject to change
without notice.

MS 9/89

BESTSELLING BOOKS
to Read and Read Again!

HOT FLASHES
Barbara Raskin
_____ 91051-7 $4.95 U.S.   _____ 91052-5 $5.95 Can.

LOOSE ENDS
Barbara Raskin
_____ 91348-6 $4.95 U.S.   _____ 91349-4 $5.95 Can.

BEAUTY
Lewin Joel
_____ 90935-7 $4.50 U.S.   _____ 90936-5 $5.50 Can.

THE FIERCE DISPUTE
Helen Hooven Santmyer
_____ 91028-2 $4.50 U.S.   _____ 91029-0 $5.50 Can.

HERBS AND APPLES
Helen Hooven Santmyer
_____ 90601-3 $4.95 U.S.   _____ 90602-1 $5.95 Can.

AMERICAN EDEN
Marilyn Harris
_____ 91001-0 $4.50 U.S.   _____ 91002-9 $5.50 Can.

JAMES HERRIOT'S DOG STORIES
James Herriot
_____ 90143-7 $4.95 U.S.

LANDMARK
BESTSELLERS
FROM ST. MARTIN'S PRESS

HOT FLASHES
Barbara Raskin
_____ 91051-7 $4.95 U.S. _____ 91052-5 $5.95 Can.

MAN OF THE HOUSE
"Tip" O'Neill with William Novak
_____ 91191-2 $4.95 U.S. _____ 91192-0 $5.95 Can.

FOR THE RECORD
Donald T. Regan
_____ 91518-7 $4.95 U.S. _____ 91519-5 $5.95 Can.

THE RED WHITE AND BLUE
John Gregory Dunne
_____ 90965-9 $4.95 U.S. _____ 90966-7 $5.95 Can.

LINDA GOODMAN'S STAR SIGNS
Linda Goodman
_____ 91263-3 $4.95 U.S. _____ 91264-1 $5.95 Can.

ROCKETS' RED GLARE
Greg Dinallo
_____ 91288-9 $4.50 U.S. _____ 91289-7 $5.50 Can.

THE FITZGERALDS AND THE KENNEDYS
Doris Kearns Goodwin
_____ 90933-0 $5.95 U.S. _____ 90934-9 $6.95 Can.

Publishers Book and Audio Mailing Service
P.O. Box 120159, Staten Island, NY 10312-0004

Please send me the book(s) I have checked above. I am enclosing
$ _____ (please add $1.25 for the first book, and $.25 for each
additional book to cover postage and handling. Send check or
money order only—no CODs.)

Name _____

Address _____

City _____ State/Zip _____

Please allow six weeks for delivery. Prices subject to change
without notice.

BEST 1/89